Spinal Cord Injury Therapy

Edited by Antonio Ibarra,
Elisa García-Vences and Gabriel Guízar-Sahagún

Published in London, United Kingdom

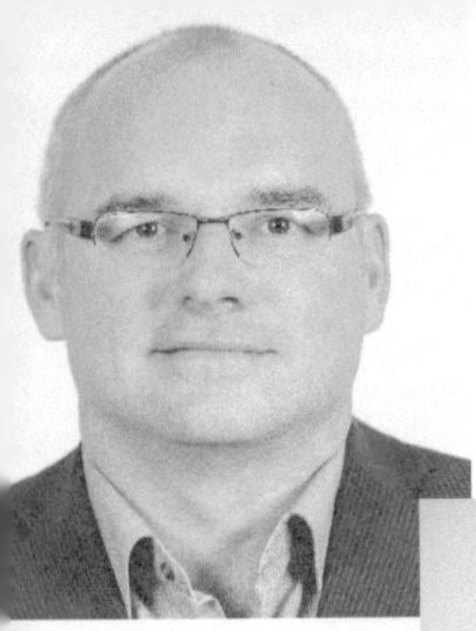
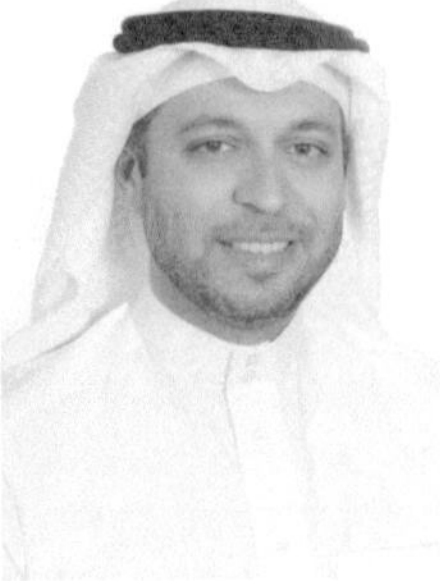
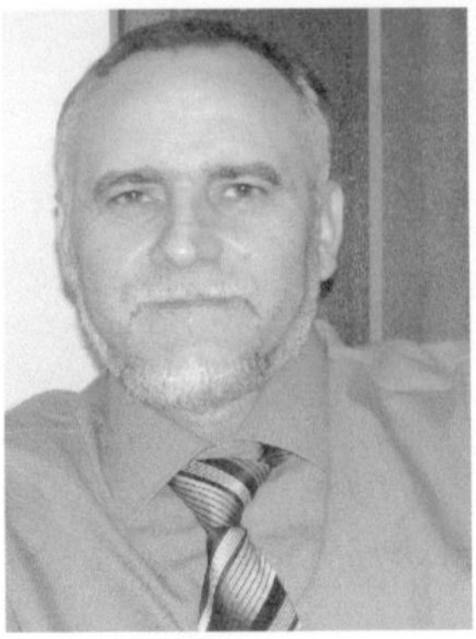
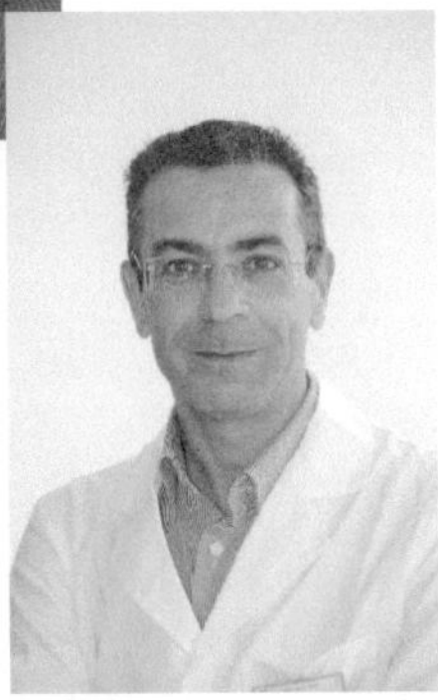
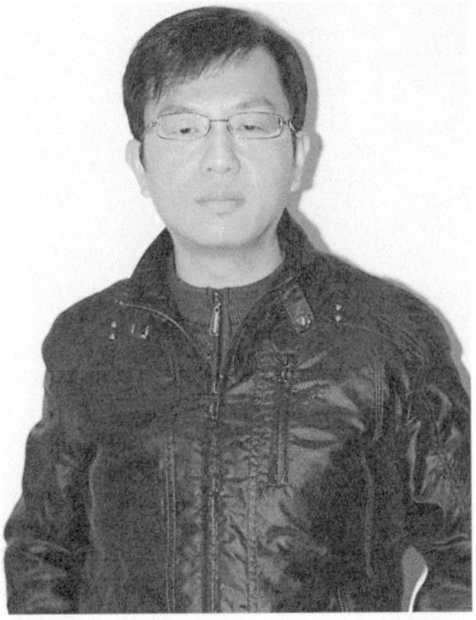
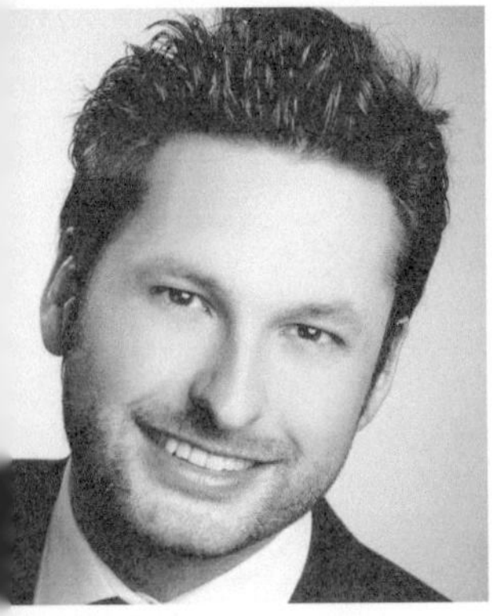
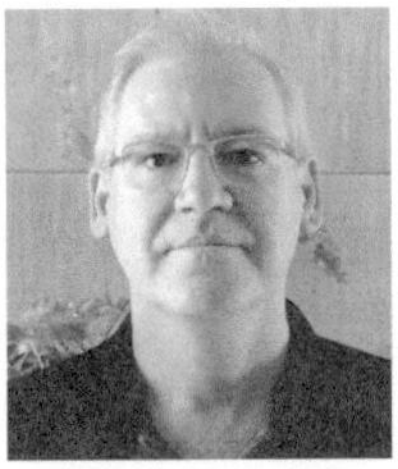

IntechOpen

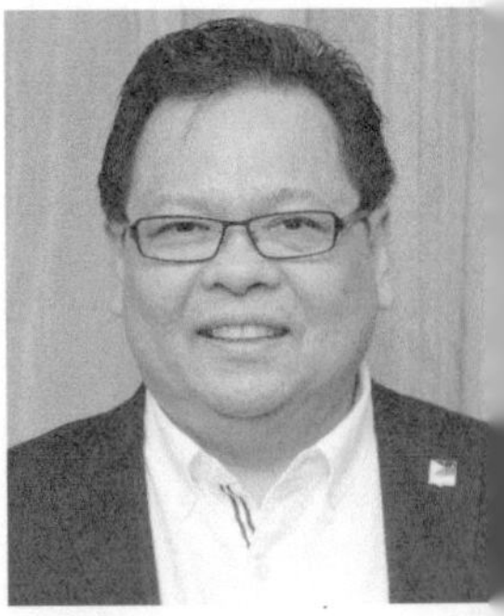
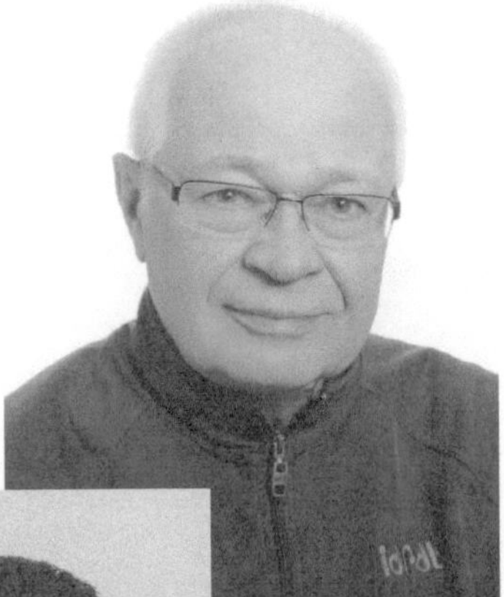
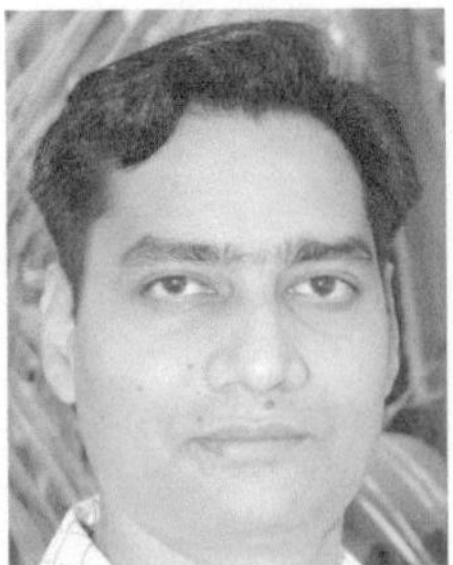
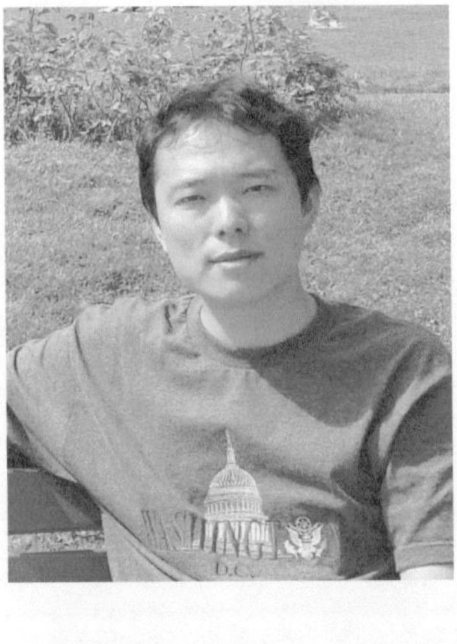
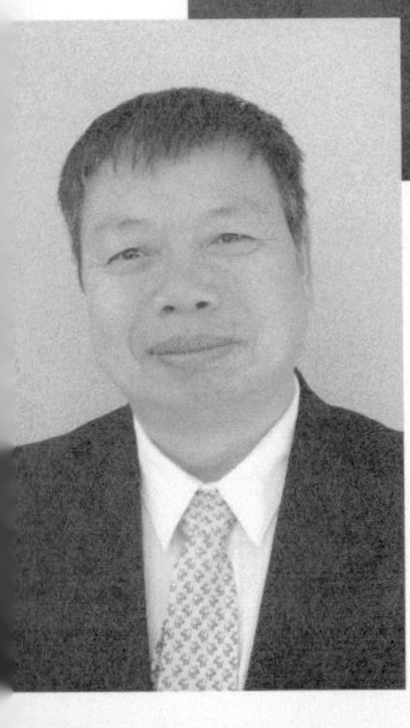
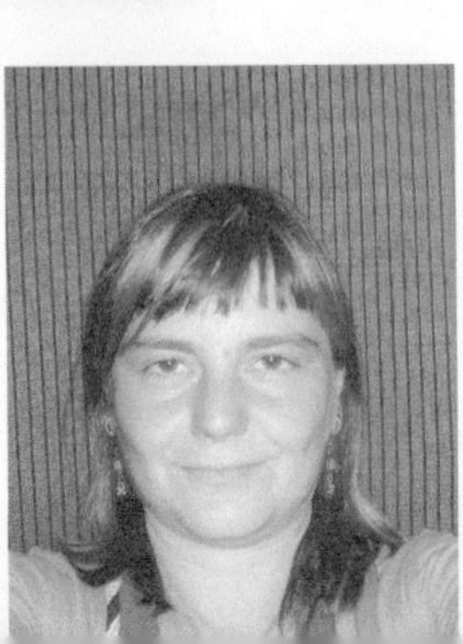

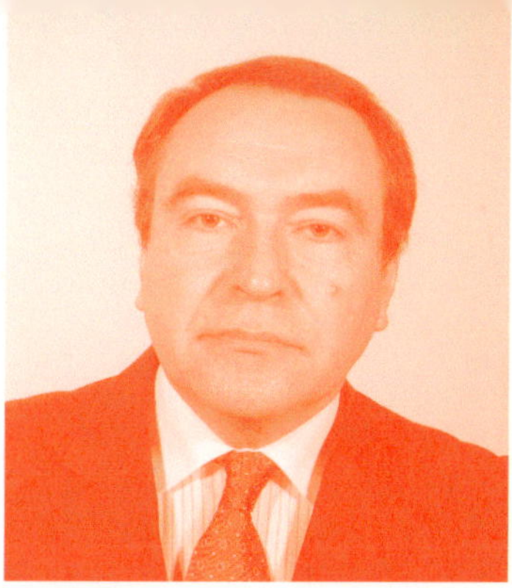
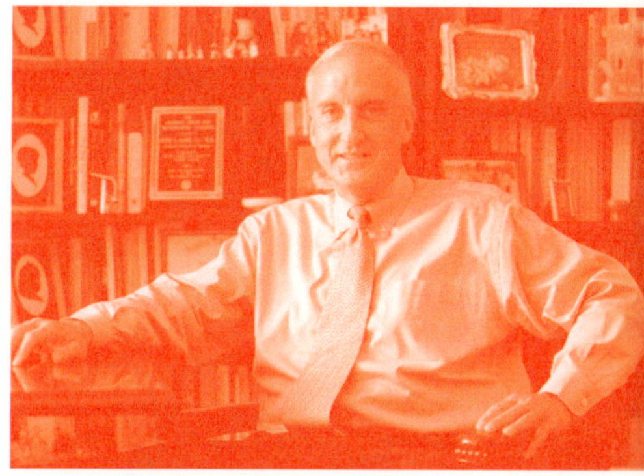
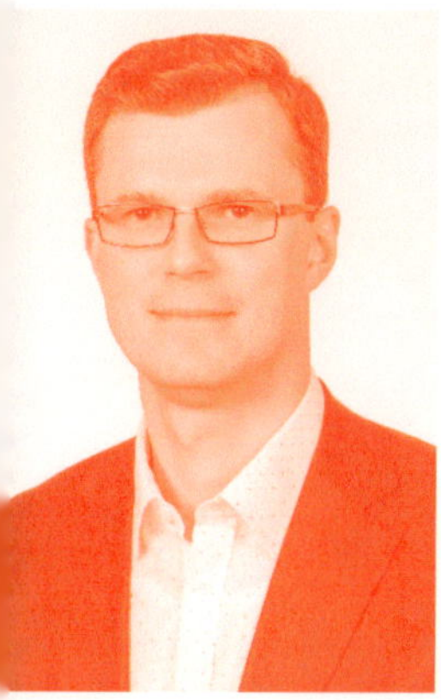
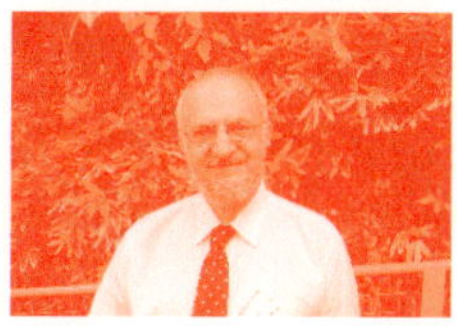
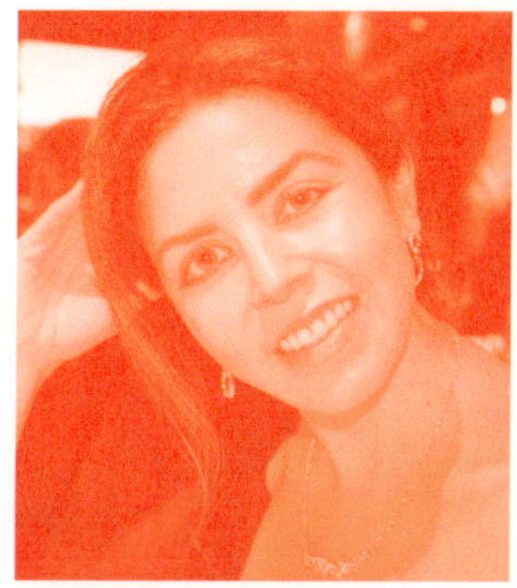

Supporting open minds since 2005

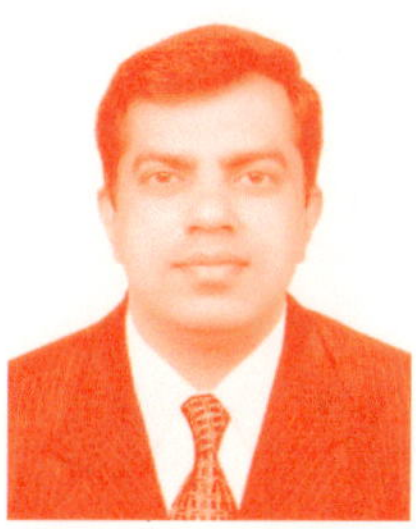
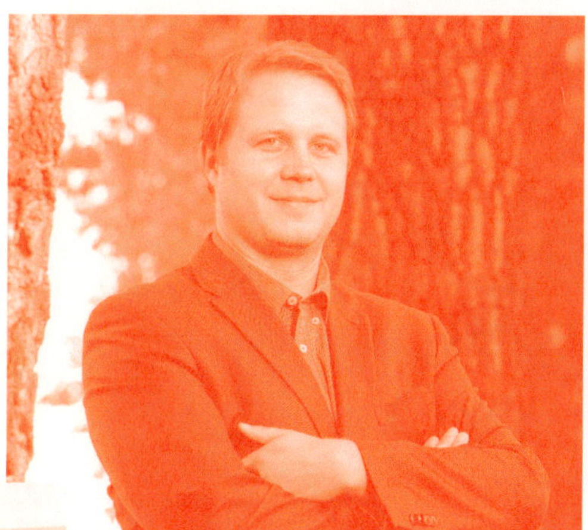
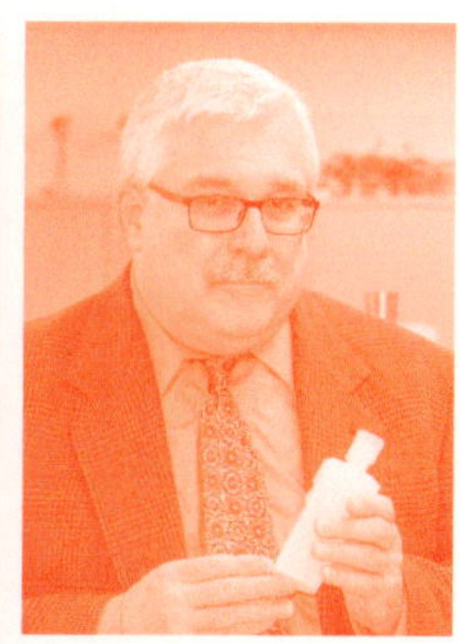
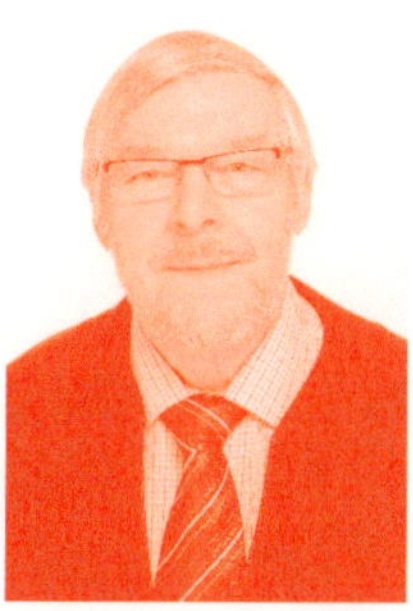
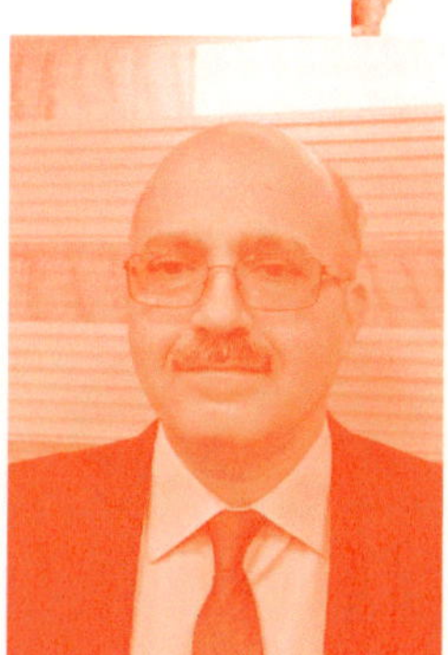
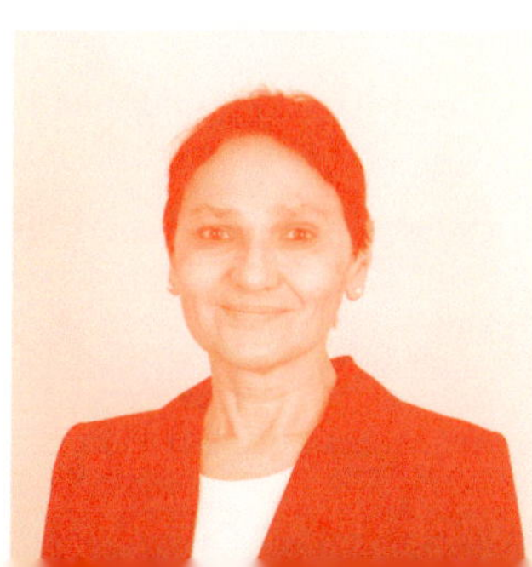
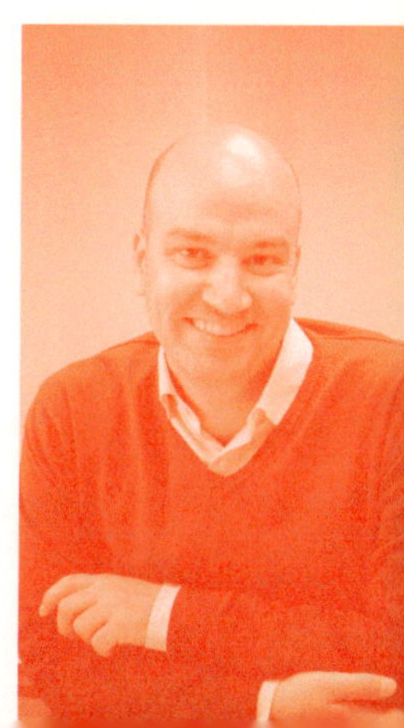

Spinal Cord Injury Therapy
http://dx.doi.org/10.5772/intechopen.77698
Edited by Antonio Ibarra, Elisa García-Vences and Gabriel Guízar-Sahagún

Contributors
Amruta Paranjape, Alok Sharma, Nandini Gokulchandran, Hemangi Sane, Prerna Badhe, Pooja Kulkarni, Vivek Nair, Susana Martiñón, Psyché Calderón-Vargas, Juan Armando Reyes-Perez, Filipe O. Barroso, Alejandro Pascual-Valdunciel, Diego Torricelli, Juan C. Moreno, Antonio Del Ama-Espinosa, Jozsef Laczko, José L. Pons, Roxana Rodríguez-Barrera, Karla Soria-Zavala, Julián García-Sánchez, Estefanía de la Cruz Castillo, Elisa García-Vences, Lisset Karina Navarro-Torres, Raúl Silva García, Jonathan Vilchis Villa, Liliana Blancas Espinoza, José Alberto Toscano Zapien, Juan Herrera García, Dulce M. Parra Villamar, Fereshteh Azedi, Mohammad Taghi Joghtaei, Soraya Mehrabi, Mohammad Ahmad, Abdualrahman Saeed Alshehri, Antonio Ibarra, Tamara D. Frydman

First published in London, United Kingdom, 2019 by IntechOpen
IntechOpen is the global imprint of INTECHOPEN LIMITED, registered in England and Wales, registration number: 11086078, 7th floor, 10 Lower Thames Street, London, EC3R 6AF, United Kingdom
Printed in Croatia

British Library Cataloguing-in-Publication Data
A catalogue record for this book is available from the British Library

Additional hard and PDF copies can be obtained from orders@intechopen.com

Spinal Cord Injury Therapy
Edited by Antonio Ibarra, Elisa García-Vences and Gabriel Guízar-Sahagún
p. cm.
Print ISBN 978-1-78984-161-9
Online ISBN 978-1-78984-162-6
eBook (PDF) ISBN 978-1-78985-844-0

For EU product safety concerns:
IN TECH d.o.o., Prolaz Marije Krucifikse Kozulić 3, 51000 Rijeka, Croatia, info@intechopen.com or visit our website at intechopen.com.

Meet the editors

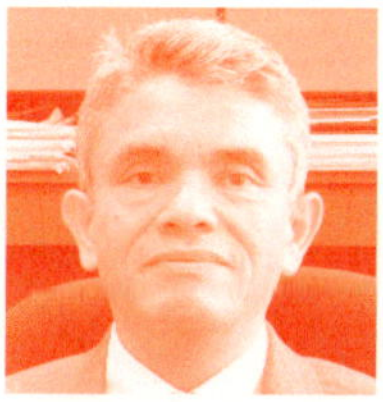

Dr. Antonio Ibarra is Head of the Health Sciences Research Center at the Anáhuac University. He earned a Masters and Doctorate in Sciences in Neuroimmunology from the National Autonomous University of Mexico. As a postdoctoral fellow in the laboratory of Professor Michael Schwartz at the Weizmann Institute of Science, and later as a scientist, he has studied the beneficial effects induced by protective autoimmunity after spinal cord injury. Dr. Ibarra has published 70 articles and 12 book chapters. His findings led him to lecture in different international meetings. He has been a reviewer of several international journals. Finally, Dr. Ibarra holds advisory academic appointments in the Anahuac University (private) and the National Autonomous University of Mexico.

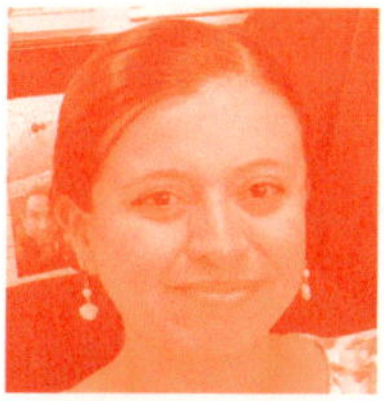

Dr. Elisa García-Vences earned her Masters and Doctoral degrees at Universidad Nacional Autonoma de Mexico. She conducted her postdoctoral training at the Instituto Nacional de Psiquiatría (INP). Dr. García was an associate researcher at INP and Instituto Nacional de Genómica. Currently, she is a professor, senior researcher, and coordinator of the Master Program on Medical Sciences at Universidad Anáhuac México. As a researcher, she is a member of the National Research System and Secretary of the Research and Bioethics Committee of the Health Sciences Research Center at Universidad Anáhuac. Dr. García has collaborated in 15 original articles on spinal cord injury, being the first author in two of them. Dr. García has participated in three book chapters as author and co-author.

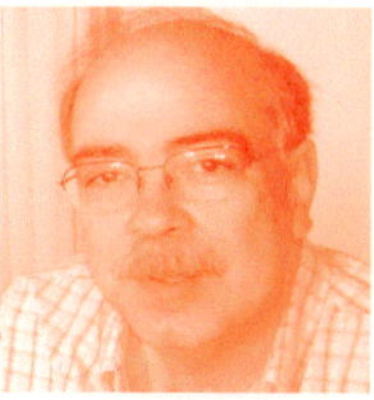

Dr. Gabriel Guízar-Sahagún is a senior researcher at the Instituto Mexicano del Seguro Social. Dr. Guízar's professional interest is basic and clinical research on spinal cord injury, mainly topics related to protection, reparative procedures, and rehabilitation. He earned his Masters and PhD degrees at the Faculty of Medicine of the Universidad Nacional Autónoma de México (UNAM). Dr. Guízar is a national research scientist and an advisor of postgraduate students from UNAM and Instituto Nacional de Psiquiatría universities. He has published 81 articles, seven chapters in books, and 92 abstracts in the memoirs of international meetings. Dr. Guízar has about 1050 citations to his scientific works, and 34 invited lectures on the topics of spinal cord injury, neural transplantation, neuroprotection, and rehabilitation.

Contents

Preface

Spinal cord injury (SCI) remains an unsolved issue when it comes to an established treatment course. To date, the focus has been on neuroprotective and neuroregeneration therapies with several options that rely on pathophysiological pathways to inhibit and enhance what is needed to establish a better microenvironment for axonal growth after an injury. This book is aimed at a discussion of the most current management alternatives in cases of SCI for a better understanding of today's perspective on the subject.

The book contains eight chapters that start with the pathophysiological picture involved in SCI and moves on to discuss therapies in depth. Chapters focusing on pharmacological agents include neuroprotective and neuroregenerative therapies. As for those concerning non-pharmacological strategies, the book contains chapters on tissue and cell transplants, scaffolds and electrical stimulation, and the combination of therapies for regeneration.

The editors would like to express their thanks to the authors of the chapters presented in this book for their invaluable contributions.

Antonio Ibarra
Coordinador del Centro de Investigación en Ciencias de la Salud,
Universidad Anáhuac México,
Campus Norte,
Huixquilucan, México

Gabriel Guízar-Sahagún
Unidad de Investigación Médica en Enfermedades Neurológicas,
México

Elisa García-Vences
Centro de Investigación en Ciencias de la Salud,
México

Section 1

Introduction

Chapter 1

Introductory Chapter: Trends in Therapeutic Strategies after Spinal Cord Injury

Tamara D. Frydman and Antonio Ibarra

1. Epidemiology

Spinal cord injury (SCI) continues to be a diagnosis without a straightforward treatment plan, even in today's advanced medical-technological time. This is a problematic pathology not only for the patient but also for the health system since, aside from causing individual disability, it also originates an important economic cost. This is due—in great part—to the age group most affected by this type of injury, which regularly involves an average age of injury of 37.1 years old [1].

Spinal cord injury can lead to fatal consequences when autonomic processes such as respiratory or cardiovascular function are altered by injury. Otherwise, the most common repercussions are those affecting motor and sensitivity skills. This generates a scenario where the patient's clinical prognosis may vary from complete paralysis to an optimum case of injury where the patient could only need physical therapy for rehabilitation [2].

The reported prevalence as of 2017 is between 440 and 526 cases per million population, with a mortality rate as high as 22% in both developed and non-developed countries [3]. Regarding its incidence, there are 130,000 new cases reported every year [4]. And even though it may not seem like a large group of patients, it accounts for more than approximately a million dollars' worth of treatment for every case reported, thus becoming an important target for research toward finding an effective treatment that can limit symptomatology as well as complications due to SCI [3].

SCI pathophysiology encompasses an important number of phenomena that mainly contribute to SC-tissue destruction and/or regeneration inhibition.

2. Pathophysiology

The understanding of the pathophysiology of acute and chronic SCI is essential to the development of new therapeutic techniques that can effectively stop damaging mechanisms and promote beneficial effects.

Primary lesion is caused by the physical consequences of injury: contusion, compression, or laceration [5]. This leads to demyelization and hemorrhage, which by itself causes ischemia and necrosis affecting nearby cells in the central nervous system. With this process comes edema which develops hours after the insult and continues to expand for several days afterward. Finally in this stage, inflammatory response, cells such as neutrophils and macrophages approach the affected area to phagocytize the apoptotic and necrotic waste [6].

IntechOpen

After this immediate response to the injury, there is a second phase with further effects on neural degeneration and tissue restoration:

- *Vascular changes*. These are due—in great part—to the ischemia that takes place, especially in the gray matter structures, and are aggravated by the hypotensive state of hypovolemia. This could be followed by a reperfusion phase that contributes to a secondary injury and the release of free radicals [7, 8].

- *Oxidative stress*. Free radicals have important effects on DNA and proteins by damaging the cell membrane through lipid peroxidation, as well as promoting apoptosis, resulting in a strong inhibition of Na-K ATPase [9, 10]. These are important consequences to keep in mind being that several treatment options available today such as methylprednisolone are related directly to this damaging mechanism [6, 11].

- *Excitotoxicity*. Glutamate, an important neurotransmitter in the central nervous system, also plays a role in the pathophysiology of SCI, as the extensive release of this molecule allows calcium entrance and the accumulation of intracellular Na and Cl (using its NMDA receptor), which in turn results in cytotoxic edema [12]. Therefore, NMDA receptor blockade becomes a therapeutic option to further explore.

- *Immune response*. As an immune-privileged site, the central nervous system is not known for having a large immune cell presence. Nonetheless, after a SCI, microglia suffers activation, and cytokines are rapidly released. There is an increase in the amount of TNF-α and arachidonic acid metabolites that can be found in cerebral spinal fluid. This, however, is a positive effect since TNF-α has been shown to increase levels of interleukin-10 which counteracts free radicals and stimulates axonal regeneration, making it a target for stimulation as a treatment option [13, 14].

- *Activation of Rho pathway*. SCI activates Rho pathway, which in turn inhibits the re-growth of axons and causes apoptosis. By inhibiting this activation, recovery improves substantially; however, there is no therapy for this purpose that has been approved yet [15].

- *Depletion of cAMP*. After injury an important reduction of cAMP in neurons occurs; this alteration inhibits neuron regeneration [16].

- *Glial scar and astrocyte activation*. The formation of a glial scar after injury represents a barrier to growing axons [17–20]. Additionally, activated astrocytes—the main cells conforming glial scar—express chondroitin sulfate proteoglycans (CSPGs) and extracellular matrix molecules like phosphocan and neurocan that, when downregulated, have shown to improve axonal regeneration, thereby proving their role in regeneration inhibition [17, 21].

At the moment, there is enough evidence about the deleterious effects exerted by each one of the abovementioned phenomena. That is why, several investigation groups are working on developing therapeutic strategies to induce neuroprotection and subsequently promote SC regeneration.

3. Neuroprotective therapies

As secondary lesion mechanisms are so abundant and have such a long-term effect on the patient's outcome; they have become the main target for SCI therapy. All of these potential treatment options are involved in various research proposals as to find suitable possibilities and improve recovery:

- *Cyclooxygenase inhibitors*. COX is a pro-inflammatory enzyme that leads to the production of prostanoids and therefore increased inflammation. This is the basis for the neuroprotective role of cox-inhibitors such as indomethacin (inhibits COX-1/COX-2 and the activity of select leucocytes, thereby preventing inflammation aggravation and edema) [22].

- *Immunophilin ligands*. These proteins are abundantly found in neural tissue and bind immunosuppressants like cyclosporine A and their analogs which are known as ligands [23]. When these ligands bind to immunophilins, they inhibit rotamase and calcineurin activity. These effects decrease immune responses such as cytokine production and neutrophil motility [24]. Ultimately, cyclosporine A binding to immunophilin slows down the demyelination process and stops the spreading of inflammation [25].

- *Antioxidants*. One of the most damaging pathophysiological mechanisms of SCI is perhaps the increased release of free radicals [26]. Methylprednisolone, currently the primary treatment for acute SCI, is aimed toward inhibiting lipid peroxidation and lactate accumulation. However, there are still concerns about it being a risk factor for pneumonia development [27].

- *Calpain inhibitors*. Calpain is a calcium-dependent cysteine protease that promotes apoptosis through enzyme degradation of cytoskeletal and membrane proteins. Researchers have found this to be associated with the increased concentration of intracellular calcium following SCI [28]. The two main classes include aldehyde-calpain and oxirane inhibitors, of this last one the primary example is E-64-d. This therapeutic option has demonstrated its neuroprotective effects in SCI models. By blocking calpains, apoptosis could be reduced [29].

- *Apoptosis inhibitors*. Caspase-3 and caspase-9 are key mediators for apoptosis after acute SCI; by inhibiting these molecules, there has been a proven clinical improvement in previous studies using minocycline. Minocycline is a second-generation tetracycline that has demonstrated to have anti-inflammatory and neuroprotective qualities in experimental studies in SCI, stroke, and neurodegenerative diseases. Talking about its antiapoptotic effects, minocycline decreases caspase 1 and caspase 3 availability, cytochrome c release, mitochondrial calcium uptake, and the release of apoptotic factors. By downsizing apoptosis in SCI, this drug reduces microglial activation [30].

- *Hormones*. Steroid hormones such as progesterone and estrogen have proven to be neuroprotective in SCI by showing decreased excitotoxicity, increased myelination, and enhanced antioxidant properties [31].

- *Na channel blockers*. Tetrodotoxin is the most investigated compound of this category; it has proven effects of better recovery by inhibiting fast Na channels and thereby lessening the continuous depolarized state of injured neurons [32].

4. Regenerative therapies

- *Pharmacological treatments*

    - *Rho pathway antagonists*. The Rho family has been associated with several pathways concerning cell proliferation, regeneration, and gene expression [33]. When activated, it leads to neurite growth blockade, especially when implicating Rho kinase (ROCK) [34]. This is why Rho-ROCK inhibitors are now under research as treatment options. These include C3 transferase, which modifies the Rho family thus minimizing its effect, and Y27632 which competes with ROCK for ATP receptors [35].

    - *Cyclic AMP enhancers*. The elevation of cyclic AMP levels is directly associated with a better neuronal response to myelin inhibitors. This has led to research for strategies that elevate cyclic AMP, for instance, the administration of dibutyryl cAMP (activating cAMP-dependent protein kinase) [36] or the inhibition of phosphodiesterase (PDE) using rolipram (a PDE-4 inhibitor that targets SNC tissue more specifically) has shown relevant effects on axonal regeneration [37].

    - *Glial scar inhibitors*. Being that the scar itself is an inhibiting factor for regeneration, several studies have tried to find a strategy to counteract this effect. Decorin is a proteoglycan molecule that has been linked to a reduction in the expression of inhibitory molecules such as brevican and neurocan as well as to the increased capability for axonal growth across myelin-rich environments [38].

    - *Hydrogels*. This type of material allows for healthy tissue to reconnect and therefore enable axonal growth across the injury. Hydrogels are usually made of hyaluronic acid or poly(2-hydroxyethyl methacrylate-co-methyl methacrylate); however, other options are being studied for their additional benefits. Some of these new prospects include poly(2-hydroxyethyl methacrylate-co-methyl methacrylate) which has shown improvement in locomotor function [39] and poly[N-(2-hydroxypropyl) methacrylamide] with evidence that it has axonogenic and angiogenic properties [40].

- *Scar removal*. Numerous research projects have proven that during chronic stages of injury (>2 weeks), there is a clear benefit when removing the glial scar given that it portrays a barrier both physically and chemically for axonal regeneration [21, 41].

- *Biocompatible matrices*. Tissucol (fibrin glue) is a fibrinogen and thrombin compound that's biocompatible and can therefore be used for cell transplant, as well as promoting growth [42]. Another alternative in this area is alginate, a biocompatible material obtained from bacteria and algae that promotes cell migration and axonal growth [43]. Other options in this category include Matrigel, polyethylene glycol, and hyaluronic acid [44].

- *Cell therapies*. In chronic stages of SCI, studies have shown that transplanting different cell types has improved recovery. Mesenchymal stem cells (MSCs) are the most promising ones so far, with the capacity to modulate the microenvironment generated after SCI by secreting anti-inflammatory molecules and switching from M1 to M2 macrophage phenotype (protective and restorer phenotype) [45]. They also release neurotrophic factors that stimulate myelination and reduce apoptosis [46].

- *Combination therapies*. As there is a large amount of experimental therapies that target different physiopathological pathways, researchers have found it to be more effective to combine some of these options when it comes to tackling acute and chronic injuries [47]. Some examples of this are the combination of several growth factors and cell transplants, combining chondroitinase ABC and physical rehabilitation and the surgical removal of scar tissue along with immune modulatory therapy [48, 49].

So far, there is no definite treatment course for patients with SCI. This fact remains, although research over the years has developed several options that target the immunologic response that is triggered after an injury and that have both beneficial and damaging consequences as well as other mechanisms such as lipoperoxidation and cytotoxicity. Hence, there are several circumstances that need to be neutralized before a second strategy can intervene that can initiate remodeling and restoring the damaged tissue. So far, the understanding of pathophysiological mechanisms has been our most powerful tool into deciphering the best therapeutic plan. Neuroprotection is the current target for pharmacological as well as non-pharmacological therapies such as rolipram, MSCs, methylprednisolone, indometh-acin, dibutyryl cAMP, and scar removal. The endpoint for all these treatment options is to encourage and enable neuroregeneration, and although as mentioned previously, there have been incredible advancements in this area, the search con-tinues for new alternatives that offer better outcomes.

Author details

Tamara D. Frydman and Antonio Ibarra*
Centro de Investigación en Ciencias de la Salud, FCS, Universidad Anáhuac México Campus Norte, Mexico

*Address all correspondence to: jose.ibarra@anahuac.mx

References

[1] DeVivo MJ, Chen Y. Trends in new injuries, prevalent cases, and aging with spinal cord injury. Archives of Physical Medicine and Rehabilitation. 2011; **92**(3):332-338

[2] Hagen EM. Acute complications of spinal cord injuries. World Journal of Orthopedics. 2015;**6**(1):17

[3] Kang Y, Ding H, Zhou H, Wei Z, Liu L, Pan D, et al. Epidemiology of worldwide spinal cord injury: A literature review. Journal of Neurorestoratology. 2017;**6**:1-9

[4] Mohit AA. Cellular events and pathophysiology of SCI. Spine. 2016;**41** (Suppl 7):S28

[5] Morales I-I, Toscano-Tejeida D, Ibarra A. Non pharmacological strategies to promote spinal cord regeneration: A view on some individual or combined approaches. Current Pharmaceutical Design. 2016;**22**(6):720-727

[6] Hayta E, Elden H. Acute spinal cord injury: A review of pathophysiology and potential of non-steroidal anti-inflammatory drugs for pharmacological intervention. Journal of Chemical Neuroanatomy. 2018;**87**:25-31

[7] Bilenko MV, Khilchenko AV. Free radical inhibitors (FRI) can prevent celigmediated LDL oxidation under ischemia (I) and reperfusion (R) of vascular wall in situ. Journal of Molecular and Cellular Cardiology. 2002;**34**(6):A10

[8] Zhang Y-S, He L, Liu B, Li N-S, Luo X-J, Hu C-P, et al. A novel pathway of NADPH oxidase/vascular peroxidase 1 in mediating oxidative injury following ischemia-reperfusion. Basic Research in Cardiology. 2012;**107**(3):266

[9] Visavadiya NP, Patel SP, VanRooyen JL, Sullivan PG, Rabchevsky AG. Cellular and subcellular oxidative stress parameters following severe spinal cord injury. Redox Biology. 2016;**8**:59-67

[10] Kwon BK, Tetzlaff W, Grauer JN, Beiner J, Vaccaro AR. Pathophysiology and pharmacologic treatment of acute spinal cord injury. The Spine Journal. 2004;**4**(4):451-464

[11] Saunders RD, Dugan LL, Demediuk P, Means ED, Horrocks LA, Anderson DK. Effects of methylprednisolone and the combination of α-tocopherol and selenium on arachidonic acid metabolism and lipid peroxidation in traumatized spinal cord tissue. Journal of Neurochemistry. 1987;**49**(1):24-31

[12] Rungta RL, Choi HB, Tyson JR, Malik A, Dissing-Olesen L, Lin PJC, et al. The cellular mechanisms of neuronal swelling underlying cytotoxic edema. Cell. 2015;**161**(3):610-621

[13] Chen WF, Chen CH, Chen NF, Sung CS, Wen ZH. Neuroprotective effects of direct intrathecal administration of granulocyte colony-stimulating factor in rats with spinal cord injury. CNS Neuroscience & Therapeutics. 2015; **21**(9):698-707

[14] Schwab JM, Zhang Y, Kopp MA, Brommer B, Popovich PG. The paradox of chronic neuroinflammation, systemic immune suppression, autoimmunity after traumatic chronic spinal cord injury. Experimental Neurology. 2014; **258**:121-129

[15] Zhou Y, Su Y, Li B, Liu F, Ryder JW, Wu X, et al. Nonsteroidal anti-inflammatory drugs can lower amyloidogenic Aβ42 by inhibiting rho. Science. 2003;**302**(5648):1215-1217

[16] Pearse DD, Pereira FC, Marcillo AE, Bates ML, Berrocal YA, Filbin MT, et al. cAMP and Schwann cells promote

axonal growth and functional recovery after spinal cord injury. Nature Medicine. 2004;**10**(6):610

[17] Fitch MT, Silver J. CNS injury, glial scars, and inflammation: Inhibitory extracellular matrices and regeneration failure. Experimental Neurology. 2008; **209**(2):294-301

[18] Jakeman LB, Reier PJ. Axonal projections between fetal spinal cord transplants and the adult rat spinal cord: A neuroanatomical tracing study of local interactions. The Journal of Comparative Neurology. 1991;**307**(2):311-334

[19] Fawcett JW, Asher RA. The glial scar and central nervous system repair. Brain Research Bulletin. 1999;**49**(6):377-391

[20] Jakovcevski I, Wu J, Karl N, Leshchyns'ka I, Sytnyk V, Chen J, et al. Glial scar expression of CHL1, the close homolog of the adhesion molecule L1, limits recovery after spinal cord injury. The Journal of Neuroscience. 2007; **27**(27):7222-7233

[21] Li X, Yang B, Xiao Z, Zhao Y, Han S, Yin Y, et al. Comparison of subacute and chronic scar tissues after complete spinal cord transection. Experimental Neurology. 2018;**306**:132-137

[22] Takeuchi K, Tanaka A, Hayashi Y, Yokota A. COX inhibition and NSAID-induced gastric damage—Roles in various pathogenic events. Current Topics in Medicinal Chemistry. 2005; **5**(5):475-486

[23] Steiner JP, Hamilton GS, Ross DT, Valentine HL, Guo H, Connolly MA, et al. Neurotrophic immunophilin ligands stimulate structural and functional recovery in neurodegenerative animal models. Proceedings of the National Academy of Sciences. 1997;**94**(5):2019-2024

[24] Ibarra A, Diaz-Ruiz A. Protective effect of cyclosporin-A in spinal cord injury: An overview. Current Medicinal Chemistry. 2006;**13**(22):2703-2710

[25] Diaz-Ruiz A, Rios C, Duarte I, Correa D, Guizar-Sahagun G, Grijalva I, et al. Lipid peroxidation inhibition in spinal cord injury: Cyclosporin-A vs methylprednisolone. Neuroreport. 2000;**11**(8):1765-1767

[26] Hall ED, Springer JE. Neuroprotection and acute spinal cord injury: A reappraisal. NeuroRx. 2004; **1**(1):80-100

[27] Martinon S, Ibarra A. Pharmacological neuroprotective therapy for acute spinal cord injury: State of the art. Mini Reviews in Medicinal Chemistry. 2008;**8**(3): 222-230

[28] Ray SK, Hogan EL, Banik NL. Calpain in the pathophysiology of spinal cord injury: Neuroprotection with calpain inhibitors. Brain Research Reviews. 2003;**42**(2):169-185

[29] Zhang S-X, Bondada V, Geddes JW. Evaluation of conditions for calpain inhibition in the rat spinal cord: Effective postinjury inhibition with intraspinal MDL28170 microinjection. Journal of Neurotrauma. 2003;**20**(1): 59-67

[30] Barut Ş, Ünlü YA, Karaoğlan A, Tunçdemir M, Dağistanli FK, Öztürk M, et al. The neuroprotective effects of z-DEVD. Fmk, a caspase-3 inhibitor, on traumatic spinal cord injury in rats. Surgical Neurology. 2005;**64**(3): 213-220

[31] Gonzalez SL, Labombarda F, Deniselle MCG, Mougel A, Guennoun R, Schumacher M, et al. Progesterone neuroprotection in spinal cord trauma involves up-regulation of brain-derived neurotrophic factor in motoneurons. The Journal of Steroid Biochemistry and Molecular Biology. 2005;**94**(1-3): 143-149

[32] Rosenberg LJ, Wrathall JR. Time course studies on the effectiveness of tetrodotoxin in reducing consequences of spinal cord contusion. Journal of Neuroscience Research. 2001;**66**(2): 191-202

[33] Kubo T, Hata K, Yamaguchi A, Yamashita T. Rho-ROCK inhibitors as emerging strategies to promote nerve regeneration. Current Pharmaceutical Design. 2007;**13**(24):2493-2499

[34] McKerracher L, Higuchi H. Targeting rho to stimulate repair after spinal cord injury. Journal of Neurotrauma. 2006;**23**(3-4):309-317

[35] Jacobs M, Hayakawa K, Swenson L, Bellon S, Fleming M, Taslimi P, et al. The structure of dimeric ROCK I reveals the mechanism for ligand selectivity. The Journal of Biological Chemistry. 2006;**281**(1):260-268

[36] Qiu J, Cai D, Dai H, McAtee M, Hoffman PN, Bregman BS, et al. Spinal axon regeneration induced by elevation of cyclic AMP. Neuron. 2002;**34**(6): 895-903

[37] Griswold DE, Webb EF, Breton J, White JR, Marshall PJ, Torphy TJ. Effect of selective phosphodiesterase type IV inhibitor, rolipram, on fluid and cellular phases of inflammatory response. Inflammation. 1993;**17**(3): 333-344

[38] Minor K, Tang X, Kahrilas G, Archibald SJ, Davies JE, Davies SJ. Decorin promotes robust axon growth on inhibitory CSPGs and myelin via a direct effect on neurons. Neurobiology of Disease. 2008;**32**(1):88-95

[39] Tsai EC, Dalton PD, Shoichet MS, Tator CH. Matrix inclusion within synthetic hydrogel guidance channels improves specific supraspinal and local axonal regeneration after complete spinal cord transection. Biomaterials. 2006;**27**(3):519-533

[40] Woerly S, Petrov P, Sykova E, Roitbak T, Simonova Z, Harvey AR. Neural tissue formation within porous hydrogels implanted in brain and spinal cord lesions: Ultrastructural, immunohistochemical, and diffusion studies. Tissue Engineering. 1999;**5**(5): 467-488

[41] Lu P, Jones LL, Tuszynski MH. Axon regeneration through scars and into sites of chronic spinal cord injury. Experimental Neurology. 2007;**203**(1): 8-21

[42] Liu J, Chen Q, Zhang Z, Zheng Y, Sun X, Cao X, et al. Fibrin scaffolds containing ectomesenchymal stem cells enhance behavioral and histological improvement in a rat model of spinal cord injury. Cells, Tissues, Organs. 2013; **198**(1):35-46

[43] Prang P, Müller R, Eljaouhari A, Heckmann K, Kunz W, Weber T, et al. The promotion of oriented axonal regrowth in the injured spinal cord by alginate-based anisotropic capillary hydrogels. Biomaterials. 2006;**27**(19): 3560-3569

[44] Preston M, Sherman LS. Neural stem cell niches: Critical roles for the hyaluronan-based extracellular matrix in neural stem cell proliferation and differentiation. Frontiers in Bioscience. 2012;**3**:1165

[45] Nakajima H, Uchida K, Guerrero AR, Watanabe S, Sugita D, Takeura N, et al. Transplantation of mesenchymal stem cells promotes an alternative pathway of macrophage activation and functional recovery after spinal cord injury. Journal of Neurotrauma. 2012; **29**(8):1614-1625

[46] Crigler L, Robey RC, Asawachaicharn A, Gaupp D, Phinney DG. Human mesenchymal stem cell subpopulations express a variety of neuro-regulatory molecules and promote neuronal cell survival and

neuritogenesis. Experimental Neurology. 2006;**198**(1):54-64

[47] Olson L. Combinatory treatments needed for spinal cord injury. Experimental Neurology. 2013;**248**: 309-315

[48] Martiñón S, García-Vences E, Toscano-Tejeida D, Flores-Romero A, Rodriguez-Barrera R, Ferrusquia M, et al. Long-term production of BDNF and NT-3 induced by A91-immunization after spinal cord injury. BMC Neuroscience. 2016;**17**(1):42

[49] Martiñon S, García E, Flores N, Gonzalez I, Ortega T, Buenrostro M, et al. Vaccination with a neural-derived peptide plus administration of glutathione improves the performance of paraplegic rats. The European Journal of Neuroscience. 2007;**26**(2):403-412

Chapter 2

Physiopathology of Spinal Cord Injury

Susana Martiñón, Juan Armando Reyes-Perez and Psyché Calderón-Vargas

Abstract

Spinal cord injuries have a multifactorial process with diverse evolution over time. An acute injury produces severe pathological and physiological changes in the organism, homeostasis is recovered, and both adverse and favorable reactions occur for the individual. In this chapter, we describe the pathophysiological follow-up to spinal cord injuries, from their acute to chronic presentations. The importance of this knowledge lies in finding solutions to the multiple disorders generated from a spinal cord injury. These will depend on the specific needs of each stage, considering the intensity of the injury, and the time elapsed from the beginning of the process until years later.

Keywords: spinal cord injury, anatomy, physiology, pathophysiology

1. Introduction

Spinal cord injury represents a devastating impairment in the patient's life that it is also known to include the patient's family. Adapting to the new condition is a challenge for all who are involved, as it is especially expensive from the economic point of view, not only for the patient and his family but also for health services, as it involves expenses of a diverse nature to offer the best quality of life for the patient. In addition, the majority of patients who suffer from it are of a productive age, which implies the need to abandon their sources of income, depending totally on their family, both financially and on their basic survival needs, such as eating, getting dressed, bathing, etc., even needing in-home specialized health care. According to various epidemiological studies, spinal cord injuries affect between 236 and 1298 patients per million inhabitants in different countries [1].

Spinal cord injury is caused by three experimental mechanisms, contusion, compression, and hemisection, all of these representing clinical lesions for study [2]. All three have different degrees of primary tissue damage; however, the three trigger severe secondary mechanisms that amplify tissue damage, hindering and even preventing the regeneration of damaged tissue. In this review, an approach is made to these destructive mechanisms after a spinal cord injury, with the aim of providing the bases of the pathophysiology of spinal cord injury to aid in decision-making for implementation of clinical and/or experimental treatments.

 IntechOpen

2. Methodology

A systematic search was conducted in PubMed and Embase with the following MeSH terms and keywords: "spinal cord injury and hemorrhagic," "spinal cord injury and secondary damage," "spinal cord injury and pathophysiology," "spinal cord injury and ischemic effects," "spinal cord injury and ionic dysregulation," "spinal cord injury and free radicals (FR)," "spinal cord injury and excitotoxicity," and "spinal cord injury and electrolyte imbalances." The search results were refined, selecting published articles from renowned journals in the medical and scientific areas that are less than 10 years old. Twenty-six studies were selected.

3. Pathophysiology of traumatic injury in the spinal cord

After a mechanical spinal cord injury (primary lesion), a series of self-destructive mechanisms (secondary lesion) is triggered that cause greater destruction of the spinal cord parenchyma with long-term sequela. Spinal cord injury is associated with mechanical damage, biochemical disorders, and hemodynamic changes [3]. The anatomic point where the primary lesion is exerted is known as the "epicenter," and the secondary mechanisms develop in a centrifugal form around the epicenter, expanding the injured area (**Figure 1**).

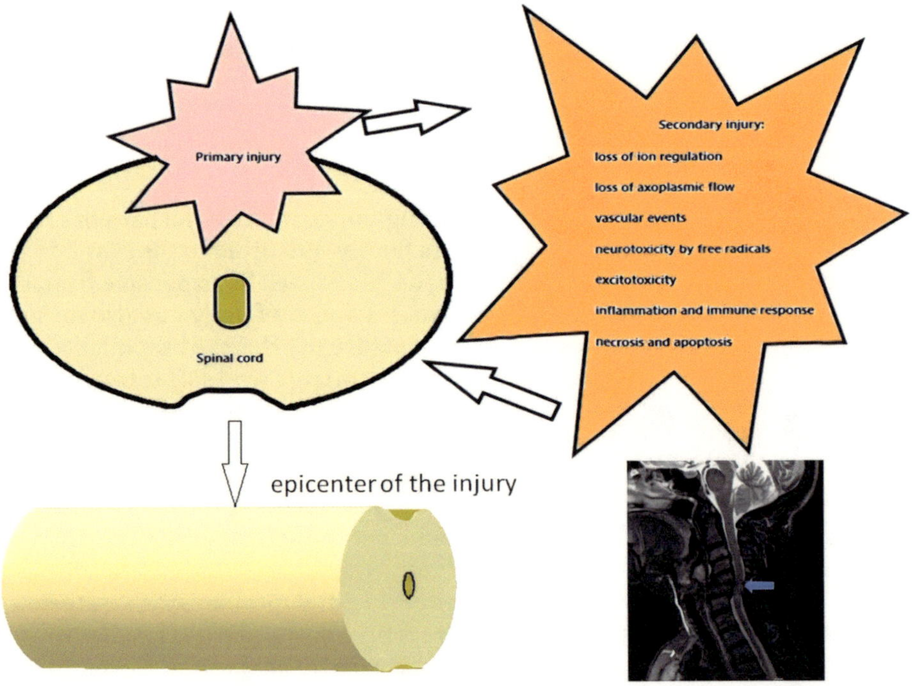

Figure 1.
Schematic summary of spinal cord injury. The primary lesion is the result of trauma directly on the neural tissue, anatomically called the epicenter of the injury to the point where the spinal cord is affected by the primary lesion; this injury triggers a series of destructive events known as a secondary injury, which will increase the area of injury in a centrifugal way, magnifying the systemic effects; these events can be observed years after the primary lesion.

3.1 Loss of ion regulation

Some of the histological changes that are observed after a TSC are the formation of edema and softening of the tissue, increase in the concentration of water, change in the caliber of the blood vessels, and rupture of the myelin surrounding the axons, in addition to a decrease in axoplasmic flow [4], with loss of ion regulation, in which an intense movement of ions is observed through an electrochemical gradient in which the concentrations of sodium (Na^+) and calcium (Ca^{2+}) increase and potassium (K^+) and magnesium (Mg^+) decrease at the intracellular level. When the gradient is altered, the electrical conduction ceases immediately, and the formation of edema is stimulated [5]. In addition, the increase in free intracellular Ca^{2+} triggers cell death by inhibiting mitochondrial function. It decreases the activation of ATP by activation of ATPase, protease, and phospholipases, with the resulting catabolism of proteins and structural lipids and inhibition of axoplasmic transport, because the increase of Ca^{2+} in the axoplasm triggers the action of neutral proteases activated by this ion and massive proteolysis of neurofilaments, which can lead to progressive collapse and fragmentation of the axon, causing tissue necrosis [6].

3.2 Necrosis and apoptosis

Activation of calpains and caspases represents other activation mechanism processes of necrosis and apoptosis by increasing intracellular Ca^{2+} [7]. The calpains constitute a superfamily of non-lysosomal proteases dependent on Ca^{2+} with a cysteine in its catalytic site. They are encoded by around 14 independent genes and have been attributed to various functions as the anchor of membrane proteins, signaling cascades, cytoskeleton remodeling, and apoptosis. The importance of caspases is the activation to start the process of programmed cell death; this has been demonstrated in deficient caspase-3 and caspase-9 mice [8].

3.3 Loss of axoplasmic flow

The axonal flow is modified because of axonal breakage. The axoplasmic flow can be retrograde or anterograde, both of which are fundamental for neuronal function. Although the cytoskeleton is composed of microtubules, actin filaments, and intermediate filaments, only microtubules are involved in the transport of materials through axons [9]. The anterograde transport is carried out through proteins associated with the cytoskeleton called kinesins, and it happens at a speed between 50 and 400 mm/day, while retrograde transport is through proteins known as dyneins [10]. The main molecules that are transported through the axons are synaptic precursor vesicles and dense core vesicles, signaling endosomes, BDNF vesicles, endosomes, late lysosomes, autophagosomes, APP, mRNA, neurofilament, and tubulin assembly and cytosolic proteins, in addition to organelles such as mitochondria [9]. Axonal fragmentation resulting from the traumatic spinal cord injury makes it impossible for the neuron to send these in both directions, which generates growth abortion and no axonal regeneration, conjointly with the formation of a fibroglial scar in the area of injury [11].

3.4 Vascular events

As mentioned earlier, the ischemic process is another mechanism through which secondary damage occurs. One of the achievements of modern vascular neurology is the description of the vascular, cellular, and biochemical changes that constitute this process [12]. The primary spinal cord injury generates a spinal cord shock, with the consequent neurogenic shock. According to Popa [13], a systemic vascular response is generated when the following are observed: coronary heart disease, arterial hypotension, and deep vein thrombosis, which may be perpetuated to become chronic processes.

Ischemic damage is constituted by the dynamic interaction between neurons, astrocytes, fibroblasts, smooth muscle, and endothelial cells that interact with the formed elements of the blood leading to cell death [12]. The main biochemical events that occur in this ischemic process are inhibition of protein synthesis, depression of intracellular energy reserves, depolarization of the cell membrane, release of intracellular K^+ followed by the release of neurotransmitters, Ca^{2+} influx to the cell, and cellular metabolic commitment, which leads to lipidic peroxidation that ultimately results in neuronal nuclear destruction and death. At the molecular level, an increase in oxygen extraction increases glucose demand, and lactic acidosis is expressed [14].

3.5 Neurotoxicity by free radicals

Another mechanism that contributes in a very important way to the increase in damage in the area of injury is the neurotoxicity caused by free radicals. These reactive molecules are powerful oxidizing agents that are in balance with antioxidant systems. They have one or more unpaired electrons due to their loss or gain, which makes them very unstable, and they are responsible for damage to cell structures of biological importance [13, 15]. The free radical species that can be found include superoxide anion (O_2^-), hydrogen peroxide (H_2O_2), hydroxyl radical (OH^-), ozone (Oz), nitric oxide (ON), hypochlorous acid (HOCl), and different metal ions. These ions are generated in the mitochondria during oxidative phosphorylation which is a process whereby ATP is formed as a result of the transfer of electrons from NADH or $FADH_2$ to oxygen through a series of electron transporters [16].

The free radical-mediated tissue injury is the result of abnormal and uncontrolled reactions of these molecules in several cellular compartments. The activity is divided into three stages: initiation, propagation, and termination [17].

The initiation of lipoperoxidation is by extraction of a hydrogen atom from the allylic carbons (=C—) of the unsaturated fatty acids of the cell membranes as well as the purine bases and pyrimidine bases of the nucleic acids, resulting in free radical alkyl (R.). Free radicals alkyl rearrange molecularly forming a conjugated diene that will react with molecular oxygen generating peroxyl radicals ($ROO^\cdot$) [18] which by extraction of one hydrogen atom from another allylic carbon, from another unsaturated fatty acid from the bilayer lipidic biological membranes reacting to hydroperoxides forms (ROOH) involving the process called propagation. Finally, the termination phase occurs by the formation of aldehydes, hydrocarbonaceous gases, and various chemical residues, including malondialdehyde ($COH—CH_2—CHO$) which will react with lipids and proteins to form conjugated Schiff bases, insoluble products that accumulate inside the lysosomes and form the pigment known as lipofuscin [19].

As will be seen below, the immune response after spinal cord injury recruits a large number of inflammatory cells, including neutrophils and macrophages, which are producers of nitric oxide. Nitric oxide is a free radical that is very important for vascular physiology since it participates in numerous regulatory events, which include vascular tone and blood pressure. This radical is formed by the reaction of L-arginine and oxygen and cofactors such as NADPH, and this reaction is catalyzed by nitric oxide synthase (NOS). Nitric oxide synthase has three isoforms: nNOS (present in brain neurons), eNOS (in endothelial cells), and iNOS (inducible in the macrophage); the first two are dependent on high concentrations of Ca^{2+} and have a physiological function, while the latter is independent of Ca^{2+} and is important in inflammatory processes [20].

Among other consequences, the alteration in the basal levels of NO produces cell death, and, although the mechanisms are not totally clear, it is known that apoptosis can occur from the inhibition of glycolysis, the Krebs cycle, and the synthesis of the DNA; also, when combined with superoxide radical, peroxynitrite is formed ($O_2^- + NO \rightarrow ONOO^-$), which is a highly reactive species and cytotoxic, as it reacts with proteins, fatty acids of membranes, and nucleic acids and decomposes into products with toxic substances that may include nitronium ion (NO_2^+), nitrogen dioxide (NO_2), and hydroxyl ion (OH^-) [16].

In this regard there are protective systems that prevent the excessive increase of oxidizing species. Among them there are three enzymes that are the most important system of this protection: superoxide dismutase (SOD), which converts the superoxide radical into hydrogen peroxide; the glutathione peroxidase, which using two molecules of glutathione in the reaction converts hydrogen peroxide into two water molecules, while the lipid peroxides are reduced in the presence of glutathione; and finally catalase, which also destroys hydrogen peroxide. However, the activity of these antioxidant enzymes is particularly low in the CNS compared to other tissues [21]. This makes this system particularly sensitive to free radicals. In addition, the CNS is rich in iron, which is the main inducer of the production of free radicals after an injury to the CNS itself. On the other hand, the cellular membrane of tissues is rich in cholesterol and polyunsaturated fatty acids which are targets of oxygen free radicals. Likewise, the CNS has few antioxidant defenses, which causes it to be even more vulnerable; in addition, studies in patients have shown that during the first year after injury, oxidative stress increases and the ability of the antioxidant defense decreases [22].

3.6 Excitotoxicity

Another mechanism of cell damage after spinal cord injury is known as excitotoxicity, caused by excessive release of neurotransmitters. A continuous increase in glutamate concentrations is observed, due to the self-amplification of glutamatergic circuits. These circuits function due to the recycling of glutamate, exocytosis of calcium-dependent synaptic vesicles, and discharge of intracellular glutamate as a result of cell lysis [23]. This abundance of glutamate, especially in a hypoxic environment, overstimulates its ionotropic receptors, N-methyl-D-aspartate (NMDA), α-amino-3-hydroxy-5-methyl-4-isoxazolepropionic (AMPA), and kainate, triggering cell death by excitotoxicity [24].

Initially, glutamate binds to its receptors and causes depolarization. This activates voltage-dependent sodium channels, causing extensive depolarization and a marked increase in intracellular sodium concentration. The chronicity of this response will lead to the release of NMDA receptors from their blockade by magnesium, leaving them available for activation by glutamate and increasing intracellular sodium. This intracellular imbalance of ions, caused by the flow of sodium, is corrected by a flow of chloride ions. In addition, this attempt to restore the osmotic balance of the cell leads to a flow of water into the intracellular space causing lysis [24]. Alternatively, excitotoxicity can kill neuronal cells by calcium-dependent mechanisms. This means that chronic depolarization leads to an intracellular calcium flux via calcium-dependent channels and the opening of channels of NMDA receptors; this flow is increased by the mobilization of calcium from its intracellular reservoirs and the reverse sodium-calcium exchange operation of the membrane, and activation of calcium-dependent self-destructive enzymes begins as a result [22].

Cell death by excitotoxicity is also observed in the glia [24], oligodendrocytes being the most susceptible cells [25]; as these cells do not have NMDA receptors, excitotoxicity is via AMPA, and kainite receptors in oligodendrocytes are more permeable to calcium in neurons, resulting in a more accelerated destabilization of their organelles; in addition, these cells have less efficient calcium buffering systems, which generate cell death in a more hasty manner [25].

3.7 Inflammation and immune response

After a TSC an intense inflammatory response is triggered that involves the action of chemical mediators, the cytokines IL-2, IL-6, and tumor necrosis factor alpha (TNF-α), and the participation of inflammatory cells such as neutrophils and mast cells. In addition to a large invasion of macrophages to the site of injury, both activated neutrophils and macrophages produce superoxide anion and nitric oxide; the latter can also be produced by platelets, endothelial cells, and microglia (CNS macrophages). Activated macrophages/microglia are important producers of cytotoxic substances, such as the proinflammatory cytokines mentioned above, causing neural damage and preventing tissue regeneration [26]. According to David [2], a flow of monocytes to the spinal cord of mice occurs at 12 hours and again at 4 days after injury. This flow is dependent on MYD88 and IL-4; however, it is not well determined whether it is from proinflammatory monocytes. In rats, researchers have been able to track dendritic cells to the area of injury by immunofluorescence, though it has not been seen in mice.

4. Discussion

The pathophysiology of spinal cord injury is not sufficiently described, and further research is needed to gain a better understanding of all the processes involved.

However, the mechanisms known so far show us a multifactorial syndrome that requires detailed study of destruction phenomena that are triggered as secondary injury. The understanding of these phenomena will lead to the rational search for solutions for patients with this condition. It is important to emphasize finding therapies that help the patient in both moments of the evolution of the lesion, as well as to provide neuroprotection, so as to favor the regeneration of injured tissue. In this chapter a brief description of the pathophysiology of the spinal cord lesion is offered in order to help the researcher find the best solutions.

There are a large number of studies with different approaches. However, a solution to all the consequences that a spinal cord injury causes has yet to be found, and so the need to find alternative treatments remains.

5. Conclusions

All the alterations and phenomena that occur at a cellular and molecular level are related to gradual degeneration of both vascular and neural tissue, destroying the anatomical substrate necessary for neurological recovery. These neurodegenerative processes cause the need to use different therapeutic strategies that reduce the damage caused by secondary injury, always looking for alternatives based on an understanding of the pathophysiology of spinal cord injury, which helps generate comprehensive and multivariable treatments that favor the recovery of function, preventing secondary damage and favoring regeneration of the neural tissue.

Acknowledgements

We thank the National Institute of Psychiatry Ramón de la Fuente Muñiz, especially QFB Ricardo J. Hernández Miramontes, and the Faculty of Health Sciences of Anáhuac University.

Conflict of interest

The authors declare that there is no conflict of interest regarding the publication of this paper.

Author details

Susana Martiñón[1,2]*, Juan Armando Reyes-Perez[3] and Psyché Calderón-Vargas[4]

1 National Institute of Psychiatry "Ramón de la Fuente Muñiz", Mexico City, Mexico

2 Anahuac University, Huixquilucan, Mexico State, Mexico

3 National Institute of Cancerology, Mexico City, Mexico

4 Centro de la Conducta S.C., Tijuana, Baja California, Mexico

*Address all correspondence to: susimar2000@yahoo.com

References

[1] Khorasanizadeh M, Yousefifard M, Eskian M, et al. Neurological recovery following traumatic spinal cord injury: A systematic review and meta-analysis. Journal of Neurosurgery. Spine. 15 Feb 2019:1-17

[2] David S, Kroner A. Repertoire of microglial and macrophage responses after spinal cord injury. Nature Reviews. Neuroscience. 2011;**12**:388-399

[3] Khaing ZZ, Cates LN, DeWees DM, et al. Contrast-enhanced ultrasound to visualize hemodynamic changes after rodent spinal cord injury. Journal of Neurosurgery. Spine. 2018;**29**:306-313

[4] Chen K, Ye J-C, Cai Z-P, et al. Intraoperative contrast-enhanced ultrasonography for microcirculatory evaluation in rhesus monkey with spinal cord injury. Oncotarget. 2017;**8**:40756-40764

[5] Pappalardo LW, Samad OA, Black JA, et al. Voltage-gated sodium channel Nav1.5 contributes to astrogliosis in an in vitro model of glial injury via reverse Na^+/Ca^{2+} exchange. Glia. 2014;**62**:1162-1175

[6] Stirling DP, Cummins K, Wayne Chen SR, et al. Axoplasmic reticulum Ca^{2+} release causes secondary degeneration of spinal axons. Annals of Neurology. 2014;**75**:220-229

[7] Cerretani D, La Russa R, Santurro A, et al. Diffuse axonal injury and oxidative stress: A comprehensive review. International Journal of Molecular Sciences. 2017;**18**:2600

[8] Auner HW, Beham-Schmid C, Dillon N, et al. The life span of short-lived plasma cells is partly determined by a block on activation of apoptotic caspases acting in combination with endoplasmic reticulum stress. Blood. 2010;**116**:3445-3455

[9] Maday S, Twelvetrees AE, Moughamian AJ, et al. Axonal transport: Cargo-specific mechanisms of motility and regulation. Neuron. 2014;**84**:292-309

[10] Brock JH, Rosenzweig ES, Yang H, et al. Enhanced axonal transport: A novel form of "plasticity" after primate and rodent spinal cord injury. Experimental Neurology. 2018;**301**:59-69

[11] Flynn KC, Bradke F, Bixby J, et al. Microtubule stabilization reduces scarring and causes axon regeneration after spinal cord injury. Science. 2011;**331**:928-931

[12] Batista CM, Bianqui LLT, Zanon BB, et al. Behavioral improvement and regulation of molecules related to neuroplasticity in ischemic rat spinal cord treated with PEDF. Neural Plasticity. 2014;**2014**:451639. DOI: 10.1155/2014/451639

[13] Sinescu C, Popa F, Grigorean VT, Onose G, Sandu AM, Popescu M, et al. Molecular basis of vascular events following spinal cord injury. Journal of Medicine and Life. 2010;**3**:254-261

[14] Zhu P, Li JX, Fujino M, et al. Development and treatments of inflammatory cells and cytokines in spinal cord ischemia-reperfusion injury. Mediators of Inflammation. 2013;**2013**:701970. DOI: 10.1155/2013/701970

[15] Popa C, Popa F, Titus Grigorean V, et al. Vascular dysfunctions following spinal cord injury. Journal of Medicine and Life. 2010;**3**:275-285

[16] Xiao M, Zhong H, Xia L, et al. Pathophysiology of mitochondrial lipid oxidation: Role of 4-hydroxynonenal (4-HNE) and other bioactive lipids in

mitochondria. Free Radical Biology & Medicine. 2017;**111**:316-327

[17] Lau A, Tymianski M. Glutamate receptors, neurotoxicity and neurodegeneration. Pflügers Archiv—European Journal of Physiology. 2010;**460**:525-542

[18] Garcia E, Silva-Garcia R, Mestre H, et al. Immunization with A91 peptide or copolymer-1 reduces the production of nitric oxide and inducible nitric oxide synthase gene expression after spinal cord injury. Journal of Neuroscience Research. 2012;**90**:656-663

[19] Scholpa NE, Schnellmann RG. Mitochondrial-based therapeutics for the treatment of spinal cord injury: Mitochondrial biogenesis as a potential pharmacological target. The Journal of Pharmacology and Experimental Therapeutics. 2017;**363**:303-313. DOI: 10.1124/jpet.117.244806

[20] Palencia G, Medrano JÁN, Ortiz-Plata A, et al. Anti-apoptotic, anti-oxidant, and anti-inflammatory effects of thalidomide on cerebral ischemia/reperfusion injury in rats. Journal of the Neurological Sciences. 2015;**351**:78-87

[21] Mohamed HRH. Estimation of genomic instability and mitochondrial DNA damage induction by acute oral administration of calcium hydroxide normal- and nano- particles in mice. Toxicology Letters. 2019;**304**:1-12

[22] Bastani NE, Kostovski E, Sakhi AK, et al. Reduced antioxidant defense and increased oxidative stress in spinal cord injured patients. Archives of Physical Medicine and Rehabilitation. 2012;**93**:2223-8.e2. DOI: 10.1016/j.apmr.2012.06.021

[23] Fernández-López B, Barreiro-Iglesias A, Rodicio MC. Anatomical recovery of the spinal glutamatergic system following a complete spinal cord injury in lampreys. Scientific Reports. 2016;**6**:1-12

[24] Fernández-López B, Valle-Maroto SM, Barreiro-Iglesias A, et al. Neuronal release and successful astrocyte uptake of aminoacidergic neurotransmitters after spinal cord injury in lampreys. Glia. 2014;**62**:1254-1269

[25] Copani A, Spampinato SF, Sortino MA, et al. Metabotropic glutamate receptors in glial cells: A new potential target for neuroprotection? Frontiers in Molecular Neuroscience. 2018;**11**:1-13

[26] Louw AM, Kolar MK, Novikova LN, et al. Chitosan polyplex mediated delivery of miRNA-124 reduces activation of microglial cells in vitro and in rat models of spinal cord injury. Nanomedicine: Nanotechnology, Biology and Medicine. 2016;**12**:643-653

Chapter 3

Reactive Astrocyte Gliosis: Production of Inhibitory Molecules

Mohammad Taghi Joghataei, Fereshteh Azedi and Soraya Mehrabi

Abstract

The astrocytic cell responses to injury have been extensively studied in a variety of experimental models, and the term "astrogliosis" is often used to describe the astrocyte reactions to injury. Cells responding in these ways to injury are often referred to as "reactive astrocytes." Glial scarring appears to be a critical feature of wound healing in the central nervous system (CNS), since elimination of the mitotically active contingent of reactive astrocytes leads to increase in the size of the wound. Reactive astrogliosis is a term coined for the morphological and functional events seen in astrocytes responding to CNS injury. The concept of reactive astrogliosis and its molecular and cellular definition in spinal cord injury (SCI) is still incomplete. Producing several inhibitory molecules discourages regeneration of axons in the injured spinal cord. This inhibition is compounded by the poor regenerative ability of most CNS axons. This is probably a more achievable therapeutic target than axon regeneration, and an effective treatment would be of assistance to the majority of patients with partial cord injuries. Of course, understanding about astrogliosis and producing mediators and inhibitory molecules such as signaling pathways help us to develop new treatment strategies for SCI.

Keywords: astrogliosis, reactive astrocyte, inhibitory molecule

1. Introduction

Astrocytes are the most numerous glial cells in the CNS, which are pivotal for various structural and physiological functions [1]. SCI triggers astrocytes to become reactive and initiate astrogliosis. Reactive astrogliosis is characterized by the proliferation and hypertrophy of astrocytes, which eventually leads to scar formation via the activation of signaling pathways such as Gp-130/activator of transcription 3 (STAT3) and transforming growth factors-beta (TGF-β/Smad) [2]. With the onset of injury, changes occur in the phenotype and morphology of astrocytes. These changes include increasing in their expression of intermediate filaments such as nestin, glial fibrillary acidic proteins (GFAP), and vimentin. Reactive astrocytes also related to the release of pro-inflammatory and anti-inflammatory cytokines such as tumor necrosis factor-alpha (TNF-α), TGF-β, interferon-gamma (IFN-γ), and interleukins (IL-1 and IL-6). It is well established that these cytokines can modulate inflammation and also secondary injury [3].

When astrocytes are activated, they change the composition of extracellular matrix (ECM) dramatically. Several ECM components including chondroitin sulfate proteoglycans (CSPGs) and tenascins are markedly upregulated in astrocytes. In addition to these phenotypic changes, astrocytes increase in number and migrate to the site of injury [4].

Therefore, astrocyte reactivity is considered as a part of endogenous mechanisms to restrict the initial tissue injury to the spinal cord and prevent extension of damage into adjacent segments. The pivotal role of reactive astrocytes particularly at first stages of SCI is indicated by recent findings. Ablation of reactive astrocytes or altering with their activation at the time of SCI injury can intensify the damage by elevating tissue degeneration and disrupt to reconstruct blood-spinal barrier (BSB) [5]. However, over time after injury, inhibitory features of reactive astrocytes overcome their constructive properties. This is mostly contributed to the upregulation of inhibitory molecules such as CSPGs that extremely prevent neuroregeneration and neural repair [6].

Astrogliosis may be heterogeneous. Not all astrocytes with the morphological characteristics of reactive astrocytes (i.e., increased GFAP) are present in areas with increased levels of ECM. Perhaps not all astrocytes that react to injury play a role in the failure of CNS regeneration, and that only those astrocytes associated with inhibitory molecules are detrimental to axon growth while those further away from the lesion may be more conducive to neurite sprouting, functional plasticity, and long-distance regeneration [7].

2. Functions of astrocytes in a healthy brain

Based on previous studies, astrocytes were for decades considered to be assisting and nurturing neurons. Regarding several studies, the protoplasmic astrocytes divide the whole gray matter of the brain and spinal cord into distinct domains, with blood vessels, neurons, and synapses contained within these domains [8], and the fibrous astrocytes are in the white matter and are in physical contact with oligodendrocytes and have an important role in myelinization; however, astrocyte functions go far beyond assistance and support [9, 10].

During development, they are considered in key developmental and postnatal traces in the CNS. Astrocytes release neurotrophic factors that regulate neuronal development, cell migration, and differentiation [11]. Developing astrocytes guide postmitotic neurons from the ventricular zone to their target destination in developing CNS. Radial glial cells, a subtype of astrocytes, guide new neurons for accurate migration [12]. Astrocytes secrete vascular endothelial growth factor that is necessary for the generation of new blood vessels in rostral migratory stream (RMS) [13]. Besides, astrocytes have connection with blood vessels through their end-feet. They can produce important mediators which contributed to vasoconstriction or vasodilation such as arachidonic acid, nitric oxide (NO), or prostaglandins [14]. Astrocytes play a critical role in the coupling of neuronal organization to signaling circuits. They are involved in hemodynamic responses with neurons through blood flow.

Astrocytes significantly contribute to the establishment and maintenance of blood-brain barrier (BBB) and BSB in the CNS [15]. Astrocytes also clear neurotransmitters such as gamma-aminobutyric acid (GABA), glycine, and glutamate from the synaptic clefts and facilitate normal synaptic transmission [16]. Astrocytes have an important function in regulation of pH in CNS. They set up proton shuttling through different proteins such as Na^+/H^+ exchanger, bicarbonate transporters acting in a sodium-dependent/independent mode, monocarboxylic acid transporters, carbonic anhydrase in both intra-and extracellular spaces, and the vacuolar-type proton ATPase [17].

Astrocytes are actively involved in the synthesis and maintenance of the ECM in the CNS. They produce a number of ECM components with both growth-promoting and inhibitory properties [18]. Astrocytes also express tenascin-C and different CSPGs with growth inhibitory properties [19]. When neuronal maturation begins in the normal CNS, CSPGs are concentrated strongly in the perineuronal nets where they are critical for stabilizing synapses and limiting undesirable plasticity [20].

3. Reactive astrogliosis in SCI

After SCI, astrocytes undergo significant cellular, molecular, and functional changes along with profound alterations in their gene expression. The reactions of astrocytes to the injury include hypertrophy of processes and soma and increasing in proliferation and upregulation of intermediate filaments such as GFAP, vimentin, and nestin. These alterations are the important markers of a phenomenon known as reactive astrogliosis [7].

Reactive astrogliosis is also indicated by high production of CSPGs, several cytokines, and chemokines such as IL-1β, IL-6, TGF-β, ciliary neurotrophic factor (CNTF), adhesion molecules, and proteins such as cyclooxygenase2, inducible NO synthase (iNOS), and calcium-binding protein S100β. These factors are considered as the functional markers of astrocyte reactivity whose levels are upregulated following CNS injuries [21].

Astrogliosis can be categorized from moderate changes in astrocytes to high reactivity related to scar formation [22]. In initial stages, there is aberrant hypertrophy of astrocytes and low upregulation of GFAP levels; however, no important proliferative activities usually occur in mild astrogliosis [23]. Mild astrogliosis or "isomorphic gliosis" is seen in the cases of axotomy, chemical lesions, or mild injury where astrocytes are distal to the site of lesion [24]. These alterations can be turned by reducing the triggering effects of upstream signaling molecules. Over time, reactive astrocytes express GFAP highly and show substantial hypertrophy, and some degree of proliferation. These remarkable expansions lead to disruption of particular regions of astrocytes and cause tissue distortion [3]. In intensive injuries, astrocytic processes overlap and become densely packed. At this stage, a glial scar encircles the epicenter of spinal cord lesion. Glial scar that is formed after local disruption of spine parenchyma is invariable and is nominated as "anisomorphic gliosis" [25].

Although astrogliosis is an early important marker of SCI in rodents, in human SCI, astrocyte reactivity is not a prominent property at acute or subacute phases, and astrogliosis seems to evolve over the time and become more evident at intermediate and chronic phases of SCI [26]. The presence of dense astrogliosis at 11 days after SCI that was still evident after 1 year post-SCI has been reported in some evidences [27]. Further investigations for astrogliosis in human SCI are necessary to examine the impact and timing. This is particularly important when translating therapeutic strategies that target astrogliosis from rodent models to human SCI.

Meningeal fibroblasts also contribute to scar formation. In fact, the glial scar formation is adjusted by a cell-cell contact mechanism between reactive astrocytes and meningeal fibroblasts at the spinal cord lesion. Signaling between ephrin-B2 on reactive astrocytes and EphB2 receptors on meningeal fibroblasts appears to carry on this process [28].

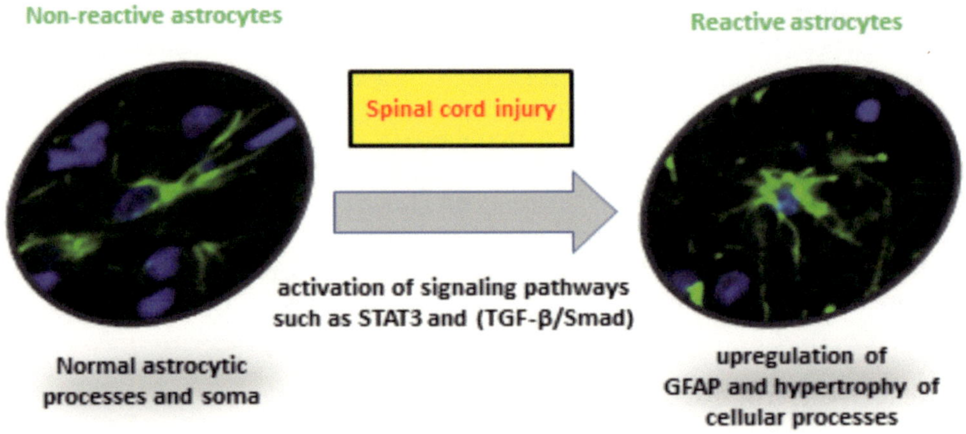

Figure 1.
Reactive astrogliosis is a response of activated astrocytes seen in spinal cord injury and can be triggered through various signaling pathways such as signal transducers and activators of transcription (STAT) and TGF-β/Smad. In most situations, it can be viewed as a defensive reaction counteracting acute stress, restoring the CNS homeostasis, and limiting the tissue damage; however, persisting reactive astrogliosis can be lead to inhibition of neural plasticity and other regenerative responses.

Reactive astrogliosis can be triggered through several signaling pathways such as signal transducers and activators of transcription (STAT) and TGF-β/Smad (**Figure 1**) [29]. Both beneficial and detrimental effects of SCI can be dependent to which signaling pathways and timing after SCI are involved. Understanding the beneficial and detrimental role of reactive astrocytes will allow us to plan therapeutic approaches.

4. Beneficial effects of reactive astrogliosis in SCI

Previously, astrocytes were known to be solely harmful in SCI, and their inhibition or ablation was considered as a therapeutic strategy. Recent studies have provided strong evidence that reactive astrocytes play pivotal roles in SCI repair with protective features [30, 31]. Repair responding by reconstructing the damaged BSB and limiting the infiltration of peripheral leukocytes and activation of resident microglia [32], modulating blood flow by the release of vasoconstrictors and regulating blood vessels diameter [33], uptaking excess glutamate, protecting neurons and oligodendrocytes from glutamate excitotoxicity, and producing antioxidants such as glutathione and defending against oxidative stress [34] are inconsiderable parts of beneficial roles of astrocytes. Reactive astrocytes upregulate the expression of intermediate filaments, GFAP, vimentin, and nestin. Interestingly, in hemisection model of SCI, double GFAP and vimentin knockout mice showed beneficial outcomes [35].

Besides, astrocytes are known to become reactive through STAT3 and suppressor of cytokine signaling 3 (SOCS3) pathways. Some evidences indicated that knockout of SOCS3 or STAT3 in GFAP-Cre or nestin-Cre transgenic models caused limited migration of astrocytes to the site of lesion and interfered with the formation of glial scar. Failure of scar formation in these animals resulted in widespread lesion [36]. Also, astrocytes can promote tissue repair and regeneration as they upregulate their expression of fibroblast growth factor-2 (FGF-2) and S100β in the injured spinal cord [37]. Furthermore, astrocyte polarity and directional migration play an important role in astrocyte ability to react to injury. Recent findings demonstrated that astrocytes depleted of the small RhoGTPase Cdc42, which is a key regulator of cell polarization, display impaired recruitment to the stab wound lesion, despite their upregulation of GFAP and hypertrophic response [38].

5. Detrimental roles of reactive astrocytes after SCI

Glial scar is a major detriment to regeneration of severed axons by upregulating a great number of molecules around the lesion and preventing regrowth of injured axons at the lesion area, including CSPGs, tenascin, semaphorin 3A, keratan sulfate proteoglycans (KSPGs), myelin-associated inhibitors, and ephrins/Eph receptors [6]. Reactive astrocytes and the ECM components generate a dense glial scar around the SCI lesion and create physical and chemical barriers on axonal regeneration. In fact, as axons come in close contact with the glial scar, they form dystrophic end-bulbs and retract without any regeneration [39]. ECM components such as CSPGs [40], tenascins [41], and collagen [42] can be act as main inhibitory factors in axonal regeneration. They could upregulate in the glial scar after SCI and obstruct axonal elongation and sprouting [43].

6. Molecular mediators of reactive astrogliosis

6.1 STAT3

STAT3 is a member of the Janus kinase STAT family and a transducer of signals for many cytokines and growth factors, such as IL-6, leukemia inhibitory factor (LIF), and CNTF [44]. The effect on astrocyte activation may be mediated via the STAT3 signaling pathway, phosphorylation, and nuclear translocation of STAT3 in astrocytes as well as indirectly through the effects of these molecules on other cell types such as microglia, neurons, or endothelial cells [45]. One of the key mediators of astrocytic scar formation after SCI is STAT3 signaling. STAT3 conditional knockout mice failed to create a glial scar that led to a widespread lesion and poor recovery of function after SCI. Lack of STAT3 activation especially led to the inability of astrocytes to move and migrate to the lesion site. This resulted in exacerbated infiltration of inflammatory cells at the site of SCI. This finding emphasized the importance of STAT3 activation in astrocytes and the impact of reactive astrogliosis in restraining leukocyte infiltration and reducing the initial insult after SCI [36].

6.2 Ephrins/Eph receptors

Erythropoietin-producing human hepatocellular (Eph) receptors and ephrin ligands have attracted considerable attention since their discovery, due to their extensive distribution and unique bidirectional signaling between astrocytes and neurons [46]. Eph/ephrin signaling is involved in the glial scar formation in CNS disorders. It has been demonstrated in a model of spinal cord injury that the development of glial scars and the exclusion of meningeal fibroblasts from the site of damage are a result of cell contact-mediated bidirectional signaling cascades, which is stimulated by the interaction of ephrin-B2 and EphB2 with reactive astrocytes and meningeal fibroblasts, respectively [28]. Another previous study demonstrated that ephrin B2 (−/−) mice exhibited a reduction in astrogliosis and an accelerated regeneration of injured corticospinal axons, which resulted in the recovery of murine motor function following spinal cord injury (SCI) [47].

6.3 TGF-β

TGF-β signaling is one of the mediators of reactive astrogliosis in SCI. TGF-β has been identified as a key trigger of CSPGs formation in the glial scar [48]. In experimental models of SCI, blockade of TGF-β signaling is shown to attenuate scar formation [49]. Interestingly, blood fibrinogen is a factor that activates TGF-β signaling after CNS injury. After vascular disruption and hemorrhage, blood fibrinogen is released into the CNS tissue, and reactive astrogliosis and CSPGs formation through the activation of TGF-β Smad2 pathway can be activated [50].

6.4 Nuclear factor-κB (NF-κB)

Activation of NF-κB transcription factor has been implicated in astrogliosis, although with some sophisticated evidence. In SCI, one study indicated that increased level of NF-κB was found in microglia/macrophages and endothelial cells but not in astrocytes [51]. However, in another study, reactive astrocytes were displayed to express NF-κB. Notably, studies in transgenic mice expressing IkBα, an inhibitor of NF-κB, under hGFAP promoter demonstrated that inactivation of astroglial NF-κB reduced the expression of TGF-β2 and CSPGs as well as other chemokines involved in glial scar formation such as C-X-C motif chemokine 10 (CXCL10) and C-C motif chemokine ligand 2 (CCL2). Moreover, blockade of NF-κB activation in astrocytes has resulted in white matter sparing and improved functional recovery after SCI [52].

6.5 Endothelins (ET)

ETs are peptides with vasoactive property. They can modulate reactive astrogliosis in various CNS diseases. ET-1 and its receptors are particularly increased in astrocytes after damage and seem to be one fundamental cause of astrogliosis [53]. In a stab wound injury, ET-1 receptor antagonist BQ788 decreased the activation and proliferation of astrocytes. ET-1 stimulates astrocyte proliferation via the activation of JNK/c-Jun signaling pathway in vitro [54].

6.6 Mitogen-activated protein kinase (MAPK)

MAPK and its downstream cascades mediate astrogliosis. It is indicated that c-mos proto-oncogene, which triggers the activation of MAPK signaling, stimulates astrogliosis. Several studies implicated the phosphorylation of extracellular signal-regulated kinase/MAPK in reactive astrocytes in mice and humans [55].

6.7 Semaphorin 3A

Semaphorin 3A (Sema3A) is an important secreted repulsive guidance factor for many developing neurons [56]. Sema3A may be secreted from non-neuronal cells such as astrocytes. Sema3A continues to be expressed in adulthood, and expression of its receptor, neuropilin-1 (Nrp-1), can be altered by nerve injury [57]. Sema3As are regarded as one of the major classes of axon repulsive molecules that lead to the failure of axons to regenerate through the neural scar. Thus, interfering with Sema3A signaling can be beneficial for axonal regrowth [58].

6.8 Aquaporins

Aquaporins may play a role in the activities of astrocytes after SCI. In particular, recent studies showed that Aquaporin-4 is critical in glial scar formation [59].

In a cortical brain injury, Aquaporin-4 null mice displayed decreased migration of astroglia as a contribution to the injury site and less glial scarring. However, findings from rat SCI indicated biphasic changes in astrocytic Aquaporin-4 levels with preliminary downregulation after SCI and a following long-lasting upregulation in subacute and chronic stages of damage. Further elucidation is needed to understand the impact of Aquaporin-4 in scar formation after SCI [60].

6.9 Components of ECM

The ECM comprises the molecules that form the structure of the matrix. There is a huge range of molecules that have been shed from the cell surface or secreted by neurons and glia [22]. Most of these shed or secreted molecules bind to the matrix to some extent, mainly to the negatively charged glycosaminoglycan (GAG) chains of the CSPGs and heparan sulfate proteoglycans (HSPGs). There are two families of cell surface-attached HSPGs, the transmembrane syndecans and the GPI-linked glypicans. Various matrix components, particularly tenascin-C and CSPGs, are upregulated in regions of CNS damage.

Tenascins are abundant in the ECM of developing vertebrate embryos. There are four members of the tenascin gene family: tenascin-C, tenascin-R, tenascin-X, and tenascin-W. Tenascin-C is the most intensely studied member of the family [61]. Tenascin-C is anti-adhesive to many forms of neuron in vitro and inhibits axon growth from many neurons, although it promotes axon growth from some embryonic neuronal types [62]. These dual properties have been assigned to different splice variants of tenascin-C and molecular epitopes within those splice variants [63].

The levels of CSPGs increase dramatically following various CNS injuries, including lesions in the spinal cord, cortex, fornix, and nigrostriatal area [20]. CSPGs are primarily generated by reactive astrocytes and to a lesser extent by oligodendrocytes and monocytes. CSPGs are a family of molecules characterized by a core protein to which the large and highly sulfated GAG chains are attached. The major CSPGs found in the CNS include lecticans (neurocan, versican, aggrecan, and brevican), phosphacan (6B4 proteoglycan), and NG2 [64].

KSPGs are another class of inhibitory ECM molecule, which are associated with spinal cord lesions [65]. Mice lacking GlcNAc6ST-1, an enzyme critical for keratan sulfate (KS) biosynthesis, have enhanced plasticity and functional recovery after SCI [66]. Recent findings show that using KS-specific degradative enzyme, keratanase II (K-II), degrade KSPGs and allow substantial motor recovery in acute phase of SCI [67].

7. Conclusion

Beneficial and detrimental effects of astrogliosis have been reported by various researches. It depends on mediators and inhibitory molecules and also signaling pathways involved in SCI. Of course, more studies about astrogliosis as a complex and multifactorial phenomenon in SCI are essential. New strategies are required to minimize the detrimental effects of reactive astrocytes for increasing their beneficial effects and improve repair and regeneration.

Limiting the amount of secondary damage done by inflammation to reduce cavitation, encouraging the production of molecules supportive of regeneration, and decreasing factors inhibiting axon growth will tip the delicate balance of growth-promoting and growth-inhibiting factors to a net environment that supports functional regrowth after CNS injury.

Conflict of interest

The authors declare that there are no conflicts of interest.

Author details

Mohammad Taghi Joghataei[1,2]*, Fereshteh Azedi[1] and Soraya Mehrabi[3]

1 Department of Neuroscience, Faculty of Advanced Technologies in Medicine, Iran University of Medical Sciences, Tehran, Iran

2 Cellular and Molecular Research Center, Iran University of Medical Sciences, Tehran, Iran

3 Department of Physiology, Faculty of Medicine, Iran University of Medical Sciences, Tehran, Iran

*Address all correspondence to: mt.joghataei@yahoo.com

References

[1] Pekny M, Pekna M. Astrocyte reactivity and reactive astrogliosis: Costs and benefits. Physiological Reviews. 2014;**94**:1077-1098

[2] Okada S, Hara M, Kobayakawa K, Matsumoto Y, Nakashima Y. Astrocyte reactivity and astrogliosis after spinal cord injury. Neuroscience Research. 2017;**126**:39-43

[3] Sofroniew M. Molecular dissection of reactive astrogliosis and glial scar formation. Trends in Neurosciences. 2009;**32**:638-647

[4] Raspa A, Bolla E, Cuscona C, Gelain F. Feasible stabilization of chondroitinase abc enables reduced astrogliosis in a chronic model of spinal cord injury. CNS Neuroscience & Therapeutics. 2018;**25**(1):86-100

[5] Faulkner J, Herrmann J, Woo M, Tansey K, Doan N. Reactive astrocytes protect tissue and preserve function after spinal cord injury. The Journal of Neuroscience. 2004;**24**:2143-2155

[6] Ohtake Y, Li S. Molecular mechanisms of scar-sourced axon growth inhibitors. Brain Research. 2014;**1619**:22-35

[7] Beckerman SR, Jimenez JE, Shi Y, Al-Ali H, Bixby JL, Lemmon VP. Phenotypic assays to identify agents that induce reactive gliosis: A counter-screen to prioritize compounds for preclinical animal studies. Assay and Drug Development Technologies. 2015;**13**(7):377-388

[8] Nedergaard M, Ransom B, Goldman S. New roles for astrocytes: Redefining the functional architecture of the brain. Trends in Neurosciences. 2003;**26**:523-530

[9] Verkhratsky A, Butt A. Peripheral glial cells. In: Glial Physiology and Pathophysiology. Hoboken, NJ: Wiley; 2013. pp. 381-433

[10] Lundgaard I, Osório M, Kress B, Sanggaard S, Nedergaard M. White matter astrocytes in health and disease. Neuroscience. 2014;**12**(276)161-173. DOI: 10.1016/j.neuroscience.2013.10.050

[11] Cahoy J, Emery B, Kaushal A, Foo L, Zamanian J, Christopherson K, et al. A transcriptome database for astrocytes, neurons, and oligodendrocytes: A new resource for understanding brain development and function. The Journal of Neuroscience. 2008;**28**:264-278

[12] Than-Trong E, Bally-Cuif L. Radial glia and neural progenitors in the adult zebrafish central nervous system. Glia. 2015;**63**(8):1406-1428

[13] Schwarz J, Bilbo S. Sex, glia, and development: Interactions in health and disease. Hormones and Behavior. 2012;**62**:243-253

[14] Schummers J, Yu H, Sur M. Tuned responses of astrocytes and their influence on hemodynamic signals in the visual cortex. Science. 2008;**320**:1638-1643

[15] Liebner S, Czupalla C, Wolburg H. Current concepts of blood-brain barrier development. The International Journal of Developmental Biology. 2011;**55**:467-476

[16] Halassa M, Fellin T, Takano H, Dong J, Haydon P. Synaptic islands defined by the territory of a single astrocyte. Neuroscience Bulletin. 2007;**27**:6473-6477

[17] Obara M, Szeliga M, Albrecht J. Regulation of pH in the mammalian central nervous system under normal and pathological conditions: Facts and hypotheses. Neurochemistry International. 2008;**52**:905-919

[18] Tom V, Doller C, Malouf A, Silver J. Astrocyte associated fibronectin is critical for axonal regeneration in adult white matter. The Journal of Neuroscience. 2004;**24**:9282-9290

[19] McKeon RJ, Schreiber RC, Rudge JS, Silver J. Reduction of neurite outgrowth in a model of glial scarring following CNS injury is correlated with the expression of inhibitory molecules on reactive astrocytes. The Journal of Neuroscience. 1991;**11**(11):3398-3411

[20] Andrews EM, Richards RJ, Yin FQ, Viapiano MS, Jakeman LB. Alterations in chondroitin sulfate proteoglycan expression occur both at and far from the site of spinal contusion injury. Experimental Neurology. 2011;**235**(1):174-187

[21] John G, Lee S, Brosnan C. Cytokines: Powerful regulators of glial cell activation. The Neuroscientist. 2003;**9**:10-22

[22] McGraw J, Hiebert GW, Steeves JD. Modulating astrogliosis after neurotrauma. Journal of Neuroscience Research. 2001;**63**(2):109-115

[23] Laywell ED, Steindler DA. Boundaries and wounds, glia and glycoconjugates. Cellular and molecular analyses of developmental partitions and adult brain lesions. Annals of the New York Academy of Sciences. 1991;**633**:122-141

[24] Ridet J, Malhotra S, Privat A, Gage F. Reactive astrocytes: Cellular and molecular cues to biological function. Trends in Neurosciences. 1997;**20**:570-577

[25] Kang W, Hebert J. Signaling pathways in reactive astrocytes, a genetic perspective. Molecular Neurobiology. 2011;**43**:147-154

[26] Norenberg M, Smith J, Marcillo A. The pathology of human spinal cord injury: Defining the problems. Journal of Neurotrauma. 2004;**21**:429-440

[27] Buss A, Pech K, Kakulas BA, Martin D, Schoenen J, Noth J, et al. Matrix metalloproteinases and their inhibitors in human traumatic spinal cord injury. BMC Neurology. 2007;7:17

[28] Bundesen L, Scheel T, Bregman B, Kromer L. Ephrin-B2 and EphB2 regulation of astrocyte-meningeal fibroblast interactions in response to spinal cord lesions in adult rats. The Journal of Neuroscience. 2003;**23**:7789-7800

[29] Gris P, Tighe A, Levin D, Sharma R, Brown A. Transcriptional regulation of scar gene expression in primary astrocytes. Glia. 2007;**55**:1145-1155

[30] Rolls A, Shechter R, Schwartz M. The bright side of the glial scar in CNS repair. Nature Reviews Neuroscience. 2009;**10**:235-241

[31] Renault-Mihara F, Okada S, Shibata S, Nakamura M, Toyama Y, Okano H. Spinal cord injury: Emerging beneficial role of reactive astrocytes' migration. The International Journal of Biochemistry & Cell Biology. 2008;**40**:1649-1653

[32] Sofroniew M. Reactive astrocytes in neural repair and protection. The Neuroscientist. 2005;**11**:400-407

[33] Mulligan S, MacVicar B. Calcium transients in astrocyte endfeet cause cerebrovascular constrictions. Nature. 2004;**431**:195-199

[34] Vermeiren C, Najimi M, Vanhoutte N, Tilleux S, de Hemptinne I. Acute up-regulation of glutamate uptake mediated by mGluR5a in reactive astrocytes. Journal of Neurochemistry. 2005;**94**:405-416

[35] Menet V, Prieto M, Privat A, Gimenez Y, Ribotta M. Axonal

plasticity and functional recovery after spinal cord injury in mice deficient in both glial fibrillary acidic protein and vimentin genes. Proceedings of the National Academy of Sciences of the United States of America. 2003;**100**:8999-9004

[36] Okada S, Nakamura M, Katoh H, Miyao T, Shimazaki T. Conditional ablation of Stat3 or Socs3 discloses a dual role for reactive astrocytes after spinal cord injury. Nature Medicine. 2006;**12**:829-834

[37] do Carmo Cunha J, de Freitas Azevedo Levy B, de Luca B, de Andrade M, Gomide V. Responses of reactive astrocytes containing S100beta protein and fibroblast growth factor-2 in the border and in the adjacent preserved tissue after a contusion injury of the spinal cord in rats: Implications for wound repair and neuroregeneration. Wound Repair and Regeneration. 2007;**15**:134-146

[38] Robel S, Bardehle S, Lepier A, Brakebusch C, Gotz M. Genetic deletion of cdc42 reveals a crucial role for astrocyte recruitment to the injury site in vitro and in vivo. Journal of Neuroscience. 2011;**31**:12471-12482

[39] Busch S, Silver J. The role of extracellular matrix in CNS regeneration. Current Opinion in Neurobiology. 2007;**17**:120-127

[40] Mizuno H, Warita H, Aoki M, Itoyama Y. Accumulation of chondroitin sulfate proteoglycans in the microenvironment of spinal motor neurons in amyotrophic lateral sclerosis transgenic rats. Journal of Neuroscience Research. 2008;**86**:2512-2523

[41] Gutowski NJ, Newcombe J, Cuzner ML. Tenascin-R and C in multiple sclerosis lesions: Relevance to extracellular matrix remodelling. Neuropathology and Applied Neurobiology. 1999;**25**(3):207-214

[42] Stichel C, Hermanns S, Luhmann H, Lausberg F, Niermann H. Inhibition of collagen IV deposition promotes regeneration of injured CNS axons. The European Journal of Neuroscience. 1999;**11**:632-646

[43] Karimi-Abdolrezaee S, Eftekharpour E, Wang J, Schut D, Fehlings M. Synergistic effects of transplanted adult neural stem/progenitor cells, chondroitinase, and growth factors promote functional repair and plasticity of the chronically injured spinal cord. The Journal of Neuroscience. 2010;**30**:1657-1676

[44] Sriram K, Benkovic S, Hebert M, Miller D, O'Callaghan J. Induction of gp130- related cytokines and activation of JAK2/STAT3 pathway in astrocytes precedes upregulation of glial fibrillary acidic protein in the 1-methyl-4-phenyl-1,2,3,6 tetrahydropyridine model of neurodegeneration: Key signaling pathway for astrogliosis in vivo? The Journal of Biological Chemistry. 2004;**279**:19936-19947

[45] Herrmann J, Imura T, Song B, Qi J, Ao Y. STAT3 is a critical regulator of astrogliosis and scar formation after spinal cord injury. The Journal of Neuroscience. 2008;**28**:7231-7243

[46] Suetterlin P, Marler K, Drescher U. Axonal ephrinA/EphA interactions, and the emergence of order in topographic projections. Seminars in Cell & Developmental Biology. 2012;**32**:1-6

[47] Ren Z, Chen X, Yang J, Kress B, Tong J, Liu H, et al. Improved axonal regeneration after spinal cord injury in mice with conditional deletion of ephrin B2 under the GFAP promoter. Neuroscience. 2013;**241**:89-99

[48] Mittaud P, Labourdette G, Zingg H, Guenot-Di Scala D. Neurons modulate oxytocin receptor expression in rat cultured astrocytes: Involvement of

TGF-beta and membrane components. Glia. 2002;**37**:169-177

[49] Davies J, Tang X, Denning J, Archibald S, Davies S. Decorin suppresses neurocan, brevican, phosphacan and NG2 expression and promotes axon growth across adult rat spinal cord injuries. The European Journal of Neuroscience. 2004;**19**:1226-1242

[50] Schachtrup C, Ryu J, Helmrick M, Vagena E, Galanakis D. Fibrinogen triggers astrocyte scar formation by promoting the availability of active TGF-beta after vascular damage. The Journal of Neuroscience. 2010;**30**:5843-5854

[51] Bethea J, Castro M, Keane R, Lee T, Dietrich W. Traumatic spinal cord injury induces nuclear factor-kappaB activation. The Journal of Neuroscience. 1998;**18**:3251-3260

[52] Brambilla R, Bracchi-Ricard V, Hu W, Frydel B, Bramwell A. Inhibition of astroglial nuclear factor kappaB reduces inflammation and improves functional recovery after spinal cord injury. The Journal of Experimental Medicine. 2005;**202**:145-156

[53] Rogers S, Peters C, Pomonis J, Hagiwara H, Ghilardi J. Endothelin B receptors are expressed by astrocytes and regulate astrocyte hypertrophy in the normal and injured CNS. Glia. 2003;**41**:180-190

[54] Koyama Y, Takemura M, Fujiki K, Ishikawa N, Shigenaga Y. BQ788, an endothelin ET(B) receptor antagonist, attenuates stab wound injury-induced reactive astrocytes in rat brain. Glia. 1999;**26**:268-271

[55] Carbonell W, Mandell J. Transient neuronal but persistent astroglial activation of ERK/MAP kinase after focal brain injury in mice. Journal of Neurotrauma. 2003;**20**:327-336

[56] Goshima Y, Yamashita N, Nakamura F, Sasaki Y. Regulation of dendritic development by semaphorin 3A through novel intracellular remote signaling. Cell Adhesion & Migration. 2016;**10**(6):627-640

[57] Sharma A, Verhaagen J, Harvey A. Receptor complexes for each of the class 3 semaphorins. Frontiers in Cellular Neuroscience. 2012;**6**:28

[58] Yamashita N, Yamane M, Suto F, Goshima Y. TrkA mediates retrograde semaphorin3A signaling through PlexinA4 to regulate dendritic branching. Journal of Cell Science. 2016;**129**(9):1802-1814

[59] Saadoun S, Papadopoulos M, Watanabe H, Yan D, Manley G. Involvement of aquaporin-4 in astroglial cell migration and glial scar formation. Journal of Cell Science. 2005;**118**:5691-5698

[60] Nesic O, Lee J, Ye Z, Unabia G, Rafati D. Acute and chronic changes in aquaporin 4 expression after spinal cord injury. Neuroscience. 2006;**143**:779-792

[61] Jones F, Jones P. The tenascin family of ECM glycoproteins: Structure, function, and regulation during embryonic development and tissue remodeling. Developmental Dynamics. 2000;**218**:235-259

[62] Brenneke F, Bukalo O, Dityatev A, Lie AA. Mice deficient for the extracellular matrix glycoprotein tenascin-r show physiological and structural hallmarks of increased hippocampal excitability, but no increased susceptibility to seizures in the pilocarpine model of epilepsy. Neuroscience. 2004;**124**(4):841-855

[63] Meiners S, Mercado M, Nur-e-Kamal M, Geller H. Tenascin-C contains domains that independently regulate neurite outgrowth and neurite

guidance. The Journal of Neuroscience. 1999;**19**:8443-8453

[64] Harris NG, Carmichael ST, Hovda DA, Sutton RL. Traumatic brain injury results in disparate regions of chondroitin sulfate proteoglycan expression that are temporally limited. Journal of Neuroscience Research. 2009;**87**(13):2937-2950

[65] Hilton B, Lang B, Cregg J. Keratan sulfate proteoglycans in plasticity and recovery after spinal cord injury. The Journal of Neuroscience. 2012;**32**(13):4331-4333

[66] Ito Z, Sakamoto K, Imagama S, Matsuyama Y, Zhang H, Hirano K, et al. N-acetylglucosamine 6-O-sulfotransferase-1-deficient mice show better functional recovery after spinal cord injury. The Journal of Neuroscience. 2010;**30**:5937-5947

[67] Imagama S, Sakamoto K, Tauchi R, Shinjo R, Ohgomori T, Ito Z, et al. Keratan sulfate restricts neural plasticity after spinal cord injury. The Journal of Neuroscience. 2011;**31**:17091-17102

Section 2

Pharmacological Therapies

Chapter 4

Current Developments in Antioxidant Therapies for Spinal Cord Injury

Jonathan Vilchis Villa, Dulce M. Parra Villamar, José Alberto Toscano Zapien, Liliana Blancas Espinoza, Juan Herrera García and Raúl Silva García

Abstract

When spinal cord injury (SCI) occurs, numerous sources of reactive oxygen species and nitrogen species may be active within first minutes or hours and even reactivate few days later. Free radical formation and lipid peroxidation (LP) have been described as an important mechanism in the beginning and accelerated progress in the development of diverse pathologies, importantly in those related to central nervous system. The compromise of molecules and cellular structures due to the oxidative state of microenvironment in SCI may determinate survival or apoptosis of resident and infiltrating cells and polarization toward an inflammatory response, which lead to an extension of damaged tissue and loss of neuronal function, or a regulatory/regenerative response. The investigation of new antioxidant agents and their action at a molecular level begins to reveal mechanisms that, if correctly modulated, promise an improvement in recovery of functions with respect to conventional pharmacological therapies. In this chapter, we will review the general mechanisms of oxidative stress and lipid peroxidation, those antioxidant treatments in experimental development and clinical phase, as well as their achievements and limitations.

Keywords: antioxidant therapy, lipid peroxidation, free radicals, spinal cord injury, nitric oxide

1. Introduction

Among the different pharmacological strategies for treating spinal cord injury (SCI), it has been observed that the quick intervention after the injury results in a better outcome for the patients [1]. This can be explained by the biochemical processes occurring at a cellular level that develop immediately after the mechanical damage, which define the subsequent physiological chain of events determining the evolution of pathophysiology of the SCI and, therefore, the degree of functional loss or recovery. One of the most important processes participating in the balance between the prevalence of damage or protection of tissue structure and the function in the central nervous system (CNS) is the generation of diverse reactive molecules by oxidative stress that target mainly lipids. This process is known as lipid peroxidation (LP), and its end products could modify proteins and DNA present in cellular structures, causing cell death and a lower probability of regeneration [2]. SCI is a highly disabling and irreversible condition that causes physiological complications (bowel, cardiac, urinary, respiratory) and it has a social-economic impact in patients. The research of new agents targeting degenerative processes such as oxidative stress and LP is important especially due to the lack of efficacy and safety of conventional therapies on patients with SCI [1]. Here, we review the efforts to discover new compounds aimed to offer an option in antioxidant treatments and the use of some in combination or in an innovative way, both in experimental and in clinical trials. We would like to mention that there is a wide range of antioxidant therapies in study, and we are only briefly mentioning some of them at this time.

2. Acute spinal cord injury mechanisms

The pathophysiology of the SCI has been divided in primary and secondary injury, the latter generally described in acute and chronic phases. The mechanisms involved in the secondary injury include biochemical degenerative processes that exacerbates damage, such as the loss of blood-spinal cord barrier (BSCB) integrity, ischemia/reperfusion, hypoxia, loss of ionic homeostasis, Ca^{2+} overload, glutamatergic excitotoxicity, immune cell invasion, inflammation, release of cytokines, free radical (FR) production, LP, and excessive production of nitric oxide ($NO^{\bullet}$). All these events occur in the acute SCI and may be clinically targeted due to their times of action, different from the unexpected primary injury [3] (**Figure 1**). It has also been demonstrated that these mechanisms are related in a way that exacerbates when the levels of oxidative stress and LP molecules are increased and that attenuates its effects when the antioxidant treatment is immediately given after SCI [4].

2.1 Mechanism of oxidative stress and free radical's generation

Reactive oxygen species (ROS) and reactive nitrogen species (RNS) are molecules that participate in oxidative stress. They are endogenously produced under physiological conditions, and in low amounts, they are essential for biological and immune process [4]. Oxidative stress could be defined as a disturbance in the pro-/antioxidant equilibrium, for the presence of high levels of ROS and RNS that exceeds the endogenous antioxidative defense mechanisms, and they are associated with damage to a wide range of molecular species, such as lipids, proteins, and nucleic acids, contributing to the pathophysiology of SCI [3].

ROS are oxygen-derived compounds that include radicals (unstable molecules with a single unpaired electron), such as superoxide ($O_2^{\bullet -}$), hydroxyl ($HO^{\bullet}$) and peroxyl ($RO_2^{\bullet}/HO_2^{\bullet}$) radicals, and non-radicals such as hydrogen peroxide (H_2O_2). Within the first minutes and hours post-injury, different sources of $O_2^{\bullet -}$ such as arachidonic acid cascade, mitochondrial leak, and enzymes systems [nicotinamide-adenine dinucleotide phosphate (NADPH) oxidase, myeloperoxidases, cyclooxygenase (COX), and xanthine oxidase], present in activated microglia and infiltrating cells (macrophages and neutrophils), may act providing $O_2^{\bullet -}$ [5], derived from the reduction of oxygen molecules (O_2) with a single electron (e^-). Although $O_2^{\bullet -}$ itself is reactive, its direct oxidative reactivity toward biological substrates in aqueous environments is relatively weak, but it distinguishes itself as an active nucleophile and oxidizing agent that can react with hydrogen donors (e.g., ascorbate and tocopherol) [4–6]. On one hand, superoxide dismutase (SOD) rapidly catalyzes the dismutation of $O_2^{\bullet -}$ into H_2O_2 and O_2 ($2O_2^{\bullet -} + 2H^+ \rightarrow H_2O_2 + O_2$), and at low pH, $O_2^{\bullet -}$ can dismutate spontaneously.

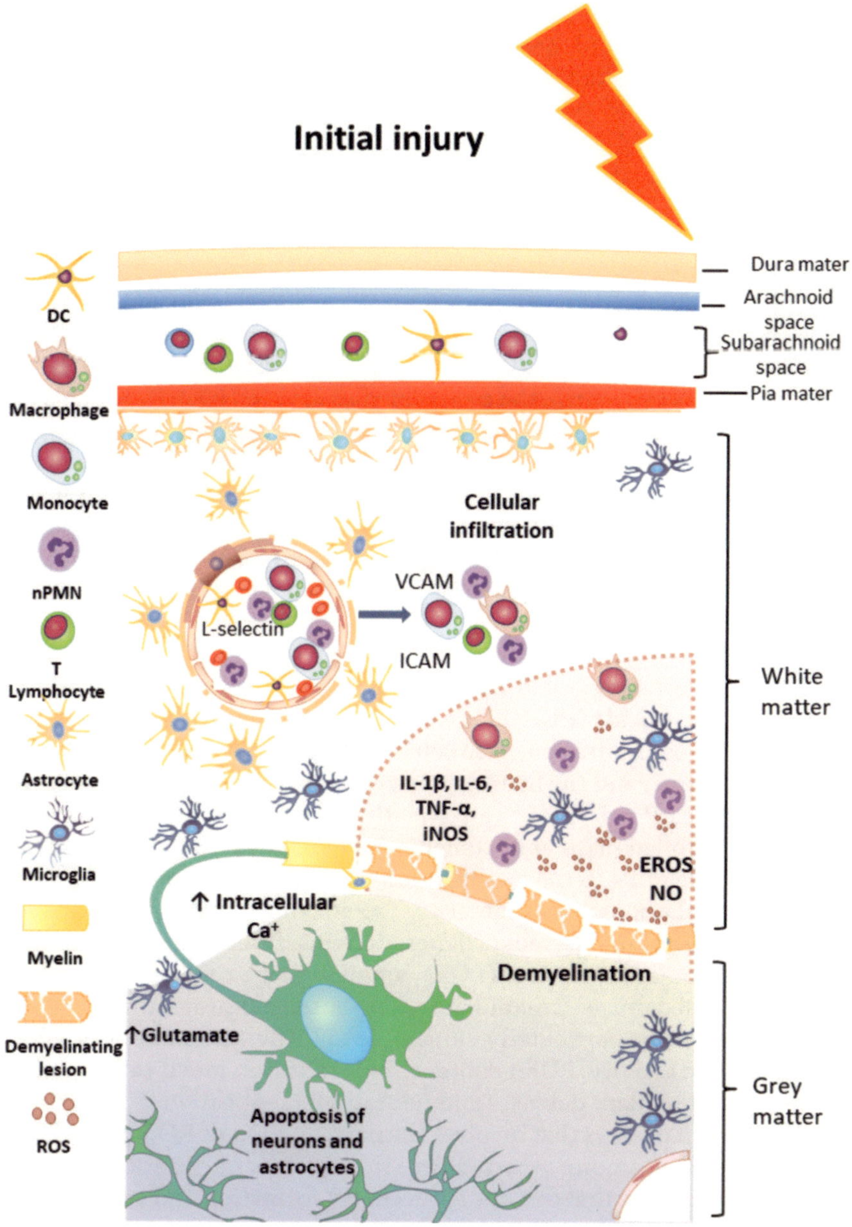

Figure 1.
Progression of the inflammatory response in spinal cord parenchyma. The condition produced by the mechanical injury induces the activation of the damage targeting mechanisms, initially propitiated by the resident microglia, which secretes pro-inflammaory cytokines. Astrocytes and endothelial cells allow the permeabilization of BSCB and express chemoattractants to facilitate the admission of immune cells from the periphery, increasing the response at site. Collateral injuries can occur, largely due to the low antioxidant capacity of neural tissue to counteract the ROS produced by inflammatory cells, spreading the damage to other uninvolved cells. The extent of the initial damage is proportional to the final capacity of the organism to recover its motor and sensory functions [155].

In oxidative stress, this H_2O_2 can react with transition metal cations to form oxidizing species such as $HO^{\bullet}$ and hydroxyl anion (HO^-), and this occurs mainly in the presence of iron (Fe) and cooper (Cu) ions. The central nervous system (CNS) is rich in ferric iron (Fe^{3+}), contained in transferrin in plasma, and ferritin intracellularly. This iron can be released from its transporters at pH values of 6 or less, like the one reached in hypoxia and accumulation of lactic acid in SCI, and become catalytic; a second source for Fe comes from the hemoglobin released after mechanical-induced hemorrhage. $O_2^{\bullet-}$ acts donating an electron to Fe^{3+}, and the ferrous iron (Fe^{2+}) catalyzes the conversion of H_2O_2 to $HO^{\bullet}$ and HO^-. Therefore, $O_2^{\bullet-}$ and H_2O_2 react in the presence of Fe^{3+}/Fe^{2+} and promote the formation of $HO^{\bullet}$ and HO^- [2].

On the other hand, $O_2^{\bullet-}$ can interact with $NO^{\bullet}$, a hydrophobic and mildly reactive radical generated enzymatically from L-arginine by nitric oxide synthase (NOS) isoforms, and give rise to one of the most important RNS, peroxynitrite $ONOO^-$ ($NO^{\bullet} + O_2^{\bullet-} \rightarrow ONOO^-$), a potent oxidizing and nitrating agent in vivo, either for direct oxidation reactions, in which it reacts with targets of low molecular weight and proteins (with thiols and metal centers), and carbon dioxide, or by derived radicals from homolytic cleavage, secondary to the reaction with carbon dioxide or protonation, included in RNS [2, 7]. Under biological conditions, $ONOO^-$ exists in equilibrium with its acidic form, the peroxynitrous acid (ONOOH), which decays rapidly by homolysis to give place to highly reactive nitrogen dioxide radical ($NO_2^{\bullet-}$) and $HO^{\bullet}$ favored by the low pH in SCI [8]. Among the different direct reactions of $ONOO^-$, one of the most relevant is this with CO_2 (from bicarbonate buffer system), to form nitrosoperoxocarbonate ($ONOOCO_2$), forming by cleavage strong oxidant agents, such as nitrogen dioxide ($NO_2^{\bullet-}$) and carbonate ($CO3^{\bullet-}$) radicals [7, 8].

2.2 Lipid peroxidation (LP)

Lipids are the most susceptible class of biomolecules to undergo oxidation; polyunsaturated fatty acids (PUFAs) are long-chain fatty acids with two or more double bonds in *cis* configuration, each separated by a methylene bridge ($-CH_2-$) at their carbon backbone, and the hydrogen attached to the methylene bridge is very easy to remove. The LP is defined as an oxidative degradation and decomposition of lipids in an uncontrolled manner by nonenzymatic pathway and occurs when ROS react with PUFAs, leading to the modification of its physicochemical properties, disrupting the cellular membrane integrity. The enzymatic pathway produces lipid mediators such as prostanoids, leukotrienes, lipoxins, resolvins, and maresins by the action of COX or lipoxygenases (LOX), among others, causing dysregulation of blood flow, BSCB damage, inflammatory response, and programmed cell death pathway [9]. The CNS is particularly vulnerable to LP by various factors: it has high oxidative metabolic activity, PUFA content, and transition metal cations. In contrast, it has low antioxidant defenses and neuron-glia replication [8, 10].

The LP is a chain process that involves the participation of ROS, RNS, PUFAs, and oxidative systems, among others, where therapeutic intervention has been proposed with molecules that can both prevent FR formation and prevent those already formed from reacting with biomolecules. Because the peak of ROS production occurs within the first 24 h after the injury, or during ischemia-reperfusion, the drugs that can be used for this "first FR production" are limited by their time of intervention. However, the phases in which LP develops may persist as long as there are oxidizable substrates, so knowing the reactions involved allows the design of strategies and drugs with a greater therapeutic window [11, 12]. The nonenzymatic peroxidation of PUFAs is the principal pathway of oxidative stress; $HO^{\bullet}$ participates as one of the starts of LP due to its solubility and the lack of an enzymatic system to eliminate it. This and other radicals remove an $H^{\bullet}$ radical inside a lipid (LH), which provides a lipid radical ($L^{\bullet}$) [11, 12] (**Figure 2**). The resonance stabilization of $L^{\bullet}$ produces a conjugated diene that reacts with O_2 to form a lipid peroxyl radical ($LOO^{\bullet}$) and generates a lipid hydroperoxide (LOOH) when it withdraws hydrogen from an adjacent PUFA, producing a second $L^{\bullet}$ [2, 12]. The LOOH are regarded as the initial product of LP, but these compounds are unstable and can be discomposed with the participation of Fe^{3+} or Fe^{2+} again in $LOO^{\bullet}$ or

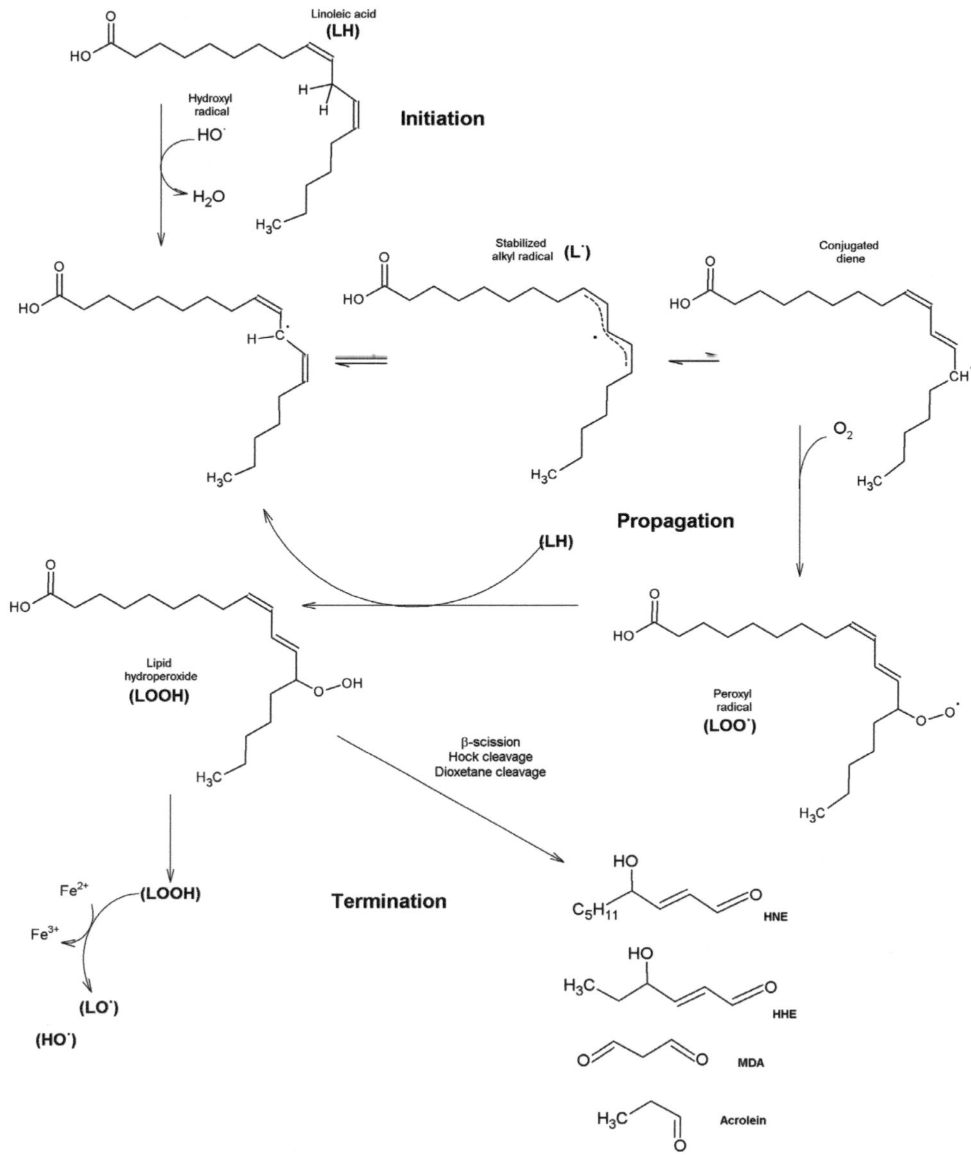

Figure 2.
The three steps of nonenzymatic lipid peroxidation of PUFAs. In the initiation step, a hydrogen atom at a bis allylic position is removed using either a radical or a redox active metal to generate a resonance-stabilized alkyl radical. The radical isomerizes to form the more stable conjugated diene, prior to reacting with molecular oxygen. In the propagation step, radicals are able to react with new substrates, forming lipid hydroperoxides (LOOH), which can react with iron creating new radicals. This step repeats until the termination step, where radicals are "quenched" by antioxidants or react with another radical. The decomposition of LOOH generates species such as MDA, HNE, etc. LH, lipid; L•, alkyl/lipid radical; LOO•, peroxyl radical; LOOH, lipid hydroperoxide; LO•, lipid alkoxyl radical; HNE: 4-hydroxy-2-nonenal; MDA: malondialdehyde; HHE: 4-hydroxy-2-hexenal. Modified from Gaschler and Stockwell [12].

alkoxyl (LO•) radicals, respectively. Both, the reduction of the LOO• to an LO• by Fe^{2+} (LOOH + Fe^{2+} → LO• + HO• + Fe^{3+}) and its conversion back to LOO• (LOOH + Fe^{3+} → LOO• + Fe^{2+}) reactions, have acidic pH optimal conditions and are more likely to occur in SCI tissue environment [5]. The LO• can initiate chain reactions too, such as the LOO• reactions describe above. Thus, one HO• can generate a high number of LOOH through a series of chain reactions. Finally, termination of chain reactions occurs by the stabilization of the radicals reacting between themselves, forming a new bond and eliminating the radical, or by donating electrons (generally $H^{\bullet}$) to the radicals by compounds, without turning into radicals. In the case of LOOH provided in the previous LP reactions, these undergo fragmentation in which oxidized PUFAs give rise to short-chain secondary products, such as hydroxy-alkenals (neurotoxic aldehydes) relatively stable like malondialdehyde (MDA), 4-hydroxy-2-nonenal (HNE), 4-hydroxy-2-hexenal (HHE), and 2-propenal (acrolein), that can diffuse within or even escape from the cell and attack targets far from the site of the original event [13] (**Figure 2**). In general, the LOOH can react in different ways that lead to a cleavage of the C-C bond and formation of hydroxy-alkenals by means of different mechanisms [13].

While the LP compromises the integrity of the cell membrane, the highly reactive secondary products can be covalently bound to proteins and DNA, compromising their structure and function. Regarding the HNE as the most studied product of LP, it must be mentioned that the HNE physiological concentration inside the cell ranges from 0.1 to 3 μM. Moreover, under oxidative stress conditions, HNE can accumulate at concentrations that range from 5 μM to 10 mM [14]. It has been demonstrated that HNE can play an important role as a signaling molecule, enhancing cellular antioxidant capacity and adaptive response at low concentrations; can promote protein and DNA damage in organelles, leading to the induction of autophagy, senescence, or cell cycle arrest; and finally can induce apoptosis or necrosis programmed cell death at a high or very high level [13, 15, 16].

2.3 Proteins as target of oxidation

The oxidation of proteins for ROS can lead to the hydroxylation of aromatic groups and aliphatic amino acid (aa) side chains, nitration of aromatic aa residues, reversible nitrosylation of sulfhydryl groups, sulfoxidation of Met residues, conversion of some aa residues to carbonyl derivatives, cleavage of the polypeptide chain, and formation of cross-linked protein aggregates. Furthermore, functional groups of proteins can react with products of LP and carbohydrate derivatives (glycation/glycoxidation) to produce inactive derivatives [17], where the irreversible protein oxidation is described by four pathways: peptide bond rupture, carbonylation, formation of protein-protein bonds, and nitration [18]. The initial oxidation can form a carbon-centered radical, which can react with O_2 to form a $ROO^{\bullet}$, to cleave protein backbone by either α-amidation or diamide pathways.

The cleavage of side chains (glutamyl, aspartyl, and probably prolyl side chains) may occur directly or by metal-catalyzed oxidation (proline [Pro], arginine [Arg], lysine [Lys], and threonine [Thr] residues), yielding carbonyl derivatives [17, 18]. One of the most important of irreversible oxidation processes is by protein carbonylation. It involves the previous protein and aa carbonyl derivatives ,$CO_3^{\bullet-}$ oxidation (reacting preferentially on tryptophan [Trp], Thr, cysteine [Cys], methionine [Met], and histidine [His] residues), ketones and aldehyde reactions over Cys, Lys, His, and by glycation/glycoxidation of Lys amino groups, etc. [2, 8, 17, 18].

The modification of the protein structure after oxidation can also give rise to intra- or inter-protein cross-linked derivatives by several different mechanisms. For example, the protein-protein bond may be due to the interaction of two carbon-centered radicals or two aromatic aa residues radicals, formed by direct attack of ROS [17]. Final products of LP, such as HNE and MDA, can cause cross-linked proteins, as reactions of both MDA aldehyde groups with two different residues in the same protein or two different proteins [17]. Another protein-protein bond is disulfide bridge (RSSR) that results from the oxidation of thiols (RSH) forming sulfenic acid (RSOH) as the last intermediate and reacting with another thiol, forming RSSR. This can be promoted in the presence of $OONO^-$ or driven by ROS and RNS, with the possibility of chain reactions [8]. Regarding this, some enzymes containing Cys, in its catalytic site, can act as scavengers, by direct interaction or consuming glutathione (GSH), due to the reversible modification of the RSSR bond [8]. HNE possess three functional groups in its structure (**Figure 2**), making this electrophilic molecule highly reactive toward nucleophilic groups such as thiol (–SH) and amino ($-NH_2$). Thus, aa such as Cys, Lys, His, and Arg are HNE targets, whose modification inhibits the functions of a variety of enzymatic and structural cellular proteins [19]. MDA with enhanced reactivity in low pH and existing as β-hydroxyacrolein is strongly reactive to nucleophiles such as Lys, His, or Arg residues [20]. Protein modifications by RNS act over aromatic, Cys, and Met residues; $OONO^-$ reacts directly with thiol groups present in a variety of proteins such as GSH, albumin, and metalloproteins (heme, myeloperoxidase, cytochrome P450, SOD isoforms, etc.) forming nitrite (NO_2^-), nitrate (NO_3^-), or $NO_2^{\bullet-}$ [8]. Finally, irreversible protein tyrosine nitration by $NO_2^{\bullet-}$, with substitution of a hydrogen in the position 3 of the phenolic ring, produces 3-nitrotyrosine (NT-3) as a specific footprint of induced cellular damage by $OONO^-$ [2, 8]. From all these modifications, diverse molecules can be identified both in cerebrospinal fluid and blood, both in humans and in animals, and they have been proposed as biomarkers to diagnose the severity of SCI. Some of those biomarkers derived from proteins are neurofilament proteins, glial fibrillary acidic protein (GFAP), tau, neuron-specific enolase, and S100 calcium-binding protein β (S100β), being part of the components of neurons, oligodendrocytes, and reactive astrocytes. A more detailed list can be found in the works of Lubieniecka et al. and the Hulme et al. review [21, 22].

2.4 DNA damage

The ROS/RNS produced in oxidative stress and LP can damage the nucleic acids of DNA; cause DNA-protein cross-links, strand breaks, and modification of purine and pyridine bases; and lead to DNA mutations. More than 20 DNA adducts have been identified, such as 8-hydroxy-2′-guanosine (8-OHdG), increased in patients in whom the antioxidant systems are suspected to be deficient [23]. MDA is an important contributor to DNA damage and mutations that can react with several nucleosides (deoxyguanosine and cytidine) to form adducts, and the major resulting product is a pyrimido-purinone called M1dG [24]. HNE can also react with deoxyguanosine to form two pairs of diastereomer adducts (4-HNE-dG 1,2 and 3,4) or etheno-DNA adducts in the presence of peroxides that could further induce DNA cross-link or DNA-protein conjugates [25, 26]. Other markers of oxidative damage in DNA, among other biomolecules, were reviewed in [23].

2.5 Enzymatic and nonenzymatic antioxidant systems

The cellular antioxidant systems are composed by antioxidant enzymes and nonenzymatic molecules able to donate electrons to different radical chemical structures. In the CNS, they are present in lower concentrations than the oxidizable substrate and are responsible of maintaining the pro-/antioxidant equilibrium, relieving oxidative stress, and reducing or interrupting uncontrolled LP, DNA mutations, protein oxidation/degradation, as well as other cell damage features. The essential endogenous components of the enzymatic antioxidant defense are SOD, catalase (CAT), glutathione peroxidases (GPx), glutathione reductases (GR), and glutathione S-transferases (GST), while the nonenzymatic antioxidants include GSH, proteins (ferritin, transferrin, ceruloplasmin, metallothionein, thioredoxin (Trx), albumin), vitamins C and E (tocopherol), trace elements, and low molecular weight scavengers, such as uric acid, coenzyme Q, and lipoic acid [4, 6, 23], which act by depleting molecular O_2 or decreasing its local concentration; removing pro-oxidative metal ions; trapping aggressive ROS, such as $O_2^{\bullet-}$ or H_2O_2; scavenging chain-initiating radicals like $HO^\bullet$, $RO_2^\bullet/HO_2^\bullet$, or $LO^\bullet$; or breaking the chain of a radical sequence [4]. There are also important exogenous nonenzymatic antioxidants (vitamins A, C, E, flavonoids, carotenoids, phenolics, acetylcysteine, exogenous selenium, zinc), acquired through diet, which are being studied. A table of these enzymatic and nonenzymatic antioxidants important in the CNS was reviewed in [23]. Preventing the formation of ROS, or at least its accumulation, and blocking or capturing those radicals already formed is the first defense against oxidative stress. The $O_2^{\bullet-}$ generated by various sources can be converted to H_2O_2 by SODs [4]. The $O_2^{\bullet-}$ intracellularly produced in the mitochondria can be converted into H_2O_2 by MnSOD (SOD3) [18]. Once generated, H_2O_2 (but not other peroxides) is decomposed to water and oxygen O_2 ($2H_2O_2 + 2GHS \rightarrow H_2O + O_2$) by the action of CAT, a ferriheme-containing enzyme. However, small amounts of ROS escape from the antioxidant defense and can be converted to $HO^\bullet$, which may be scavenged by low molecular mass nonenzymatic antioxidants, such as ascorbate, tocopherol, GSH, etc. [27]. H_2O_2 is also reduced by the action of different peroxidases, such as GPx ($H_2O_2 + 2GHS \rightarrow H_2O + GSSG$), which, additionally, can reduce lipid hydroperoxides ($LOOH + 2GSH \rightarrow LOH + GSSG$) [11, 12]. Other enzymes that catalyze this reaction include peroxiredoxin and thioredoxin reductase [4]. Some enzymes that participate in the detoxification of LP products by oxidation, reduction, and glutathione conjugation, the latter being a mechanism also used to reverse the effects of RNS, are aldehyde dehydrogenases (ALDH), alcohol dehydrogenase (ADH), aldo-keto reductase (AKR), and the aforementioned GST, GPx, and GR [28].

In SCI, the primary injury causes disruption of blood flow and vascular insult, such as ischemia-reperfusion, which conducts to the loss of metabolic function of cells in gray matter with decrease of ATP, causing depolarization of membranes due to the inhibition of Na^+/K^+ and Ca^{2+} ATPases function. Ca^{2+} overload and glutamate excitotoxicity compromise the function and integrity of mitochondria through the activation of proteases and inactivation of important enzymes. Due to the low ratio of antioxidant systems' oxidizable substrate in acute SCI, the mitochondrial antioxidant reserves decrease and are incapable of restoring the redox equilibrium, giving place to an increase of mitochondrial concentration of $O_2^{\bullet-}$ and an increase and leak of free radicals formed downstream including $ONOO^-$, initiating LP. The damage produced by this excess of radicals or end products of LP over proteins and membranes of the mitochondria and endoplasmic reticulum potentiates the processes of secondary injury mentioned here to the local and adjacent cells to SCI [4].

3. Antioxidant therapy strategies

The early therapeutic intervention for SCI is crucial to improve the chances of maximum possible recovery. This was observed in clinical trials where the current treatment of choice, methylprednisolone sodium succinate (MP or MPSS), was effective only when administered within the first 8 h after injury, at high doses (5.4 mg/kg/h). In 48-h regimens, however, it increases the incidence of complications from infections (severe sepsis and pneumonia), while the 24-h safe regimen is not effective in the long term, at least after 3 h [1]. Being an ineffective treatment, there are no alternative therapeutic treatments that offer safety and certainty regarding the recovery of the motor function. The research of new pharmacological agents for the treatment of SCI focuses on the processes of secondary injury, being antioxidant therapies the most important. The main goals of drug therapies for SCI can be classified in neuroprotection and neuroregeneration; antioxidant therapies are cataloged within the first. Here we present some of the agents that are in experimental phase and others when mentioned, in clinical trials, either because their efficacy has been demonstrated in animal models or because of their use already approved in other pathologies. Regarding the diverse SCI models, they have been used to simulate SCI with high relevance and validity to preclinical evaluation due to the replication of human traumatic injuries. The rational use of animals is strongly controlled, and the possibility of pain and distress must be considered and minimized by veterinary staff through the appropriate use of analgesics and animal care.

3.1 Melatonin

Melatonin (N-acetyl-5-methoxytryptamine) is a pleiotropic compound that works mainly in the regulation of circadian rhythms and sleep. When reacting with ROS, such as HO^-, $H_2O^{\bullet}$, and $LOO^{\bullet}$, it is converted to cyclic 3-hydroxymelatonin. It stimulates the expression and activity of SOD, GPx, CAT, and GR and inhibits or decreases the expression of pro-oxidative NOs, different signaling pathways, transcription factors, and pro-inflammatory cytokines [29–31]. Decreased melatonin production has been linked to various CNS disorders, and the neuroprotective activity was detected in rat models of traumatic brain injury ischemic stroke and SCI [29, 30]. To cite only some SCI examples, in a study in Sprague-Dawley rats of 250 g with moderate lesion, 10 mg/kg of melatonin was applied subcutaneously twice a day for 4 weeks, and an increase in motor recovery and decrease in inducible nitric oxide synthase (iNOS) expression were observed. Intravenously, it decreased the synthesis of MDA and increased the synthesis of GSH and angiopoietin 1, and in mice with severe lesion, it decreased the expression of interleukin 1 beta (IL-1β) and NG-2 (neuron/glial antigen 2) [30, 32, 33]. In a model with lesion with vascular clips, the administration of 30 mg/kg alleviated post-traumatic injury associated with SCI by binding the PPARα-receptor; the administration of 50 mg/kg in moderate lesion decreased the BSCB permeability modulating the expression of brain-derived neurotrophic factor (BDNF), growth-associated protein 43 (GAP-43), and caspase-3 [33–35]. In combination therapy with dexamethasone (10–0.025 mg/kg), it showed significant anti-inflammatory effects, attenuating the synthesis of tumor necrosis factor alpha (TNF-α) and iNOS and the nitration of tyrosine residues, increasing tissue recovery and motor capacity in an experimental SCI model of mouse [36], while the combination with methylprednisolone favored neurological recovery and decreased LP; its administration with zinc activated the internal antioxidant system and also decreased the LP [37–39].

3.2 Minocycline

Minocycline hydrochloride is an available semisynthetic tetracycline antibiotic with potent anti-inflammatory (regulation of phospholipase A_2 and MAPK/PIK3 pathways) and neuroprotective (protecting against glutamate-induced inflammation) activities; it also inhibits matrix metalloproteinases and mitochondrial Ca^{2+} influx. Minocycline has antioxidant and antiapoptotic properties, probably acting at high doses as a direct radical scavenger, like vitamin E, due to its phenolic ring structure [40]. In rats with SCI, minocycline given at oral doses of 3, 30, and 90 mg/kg 1 and 24 h after the lesion reduced MDA concentration and increased

GPx and SOD activity in a dose-dependent manner [41]. Minocycline decreased pro-inflammatory cytokines and the chemokines release from microglia and their activation, including their levels of enzymes that regulate LP and NO production [42]. A recovery difference between treatment and placebo, approaching to statistical significance in patients with cervical injury, was shown in a phase II clinical trial. The trail determined safety and dose optimization, within 12 h of SCI and for 7 days, with steady-state concentrations of 12.7 μg/mL in serum and 2.3 μg/mL in in cerebrospinal fluid (ClinicalTrials.gov number NCT00559494) [43].

3.3 Estrogen

Treatment with gonadal steroid hormones (estradiol, testosterone, estrogen) has resulted in motor recovery with a reduction of the lesion volume in animal models. Through its receptors (ERα and ERβ), estrogen exerts neuroprotection at physiological concentrations, and it exerts better neuroprotection as an antioxidant at high concentrations. Estrogen modulates gene expression; promotes angiogenesis; inhibits inflammation, blocking microglia from releasing inflammatory molecules such as TNF-α, ROS, prostaglandin E_2, etc.; regulates the expression of antioxidant enzymes; and induces mitochondrial GSH production [44]. Different low doses and times of administration (between 10 and 100 μg/kg/day/7 days to 4 mg/kg/15 min and 24 h, i.v.) appear to be effective, suggesting that pre-treatment or immediate posttreatment at either physiological or supraphysiological dose could minimize secondary injury in SCI and promote functional recovery, reflected in both acute and chronic stages [44, 45]. Additionally, the development of selective agonists of ER with higher affinity for ERα, ERβ, or both, such as tamoxifen, looks promising in SCI treatment, when applied in subdermal implants 7 days before, immediately, or 24 h post-injury; with an immediate release of 0.71 mg/day for 21 days, it provided motor recovery and preservation of white matter, dorsal and ventral horn neurons, with a decrease of $O_2^{\bullet-}$ production [46].

3.4 Omega-3 fatty acids

The omega-3 fatty acids: α-linolenic acid, eicosapentaenoic acid (EPA, with five unsaturated bonds), and docosahexaenoic acid (DHA, with six unsaturated bonds) are part of the triacylglycerols that are consumed in the diet. DHA is a primary structural component of human brain, cerebral cortex, and retina. The lack of DHA may affect the fluidity and integrity of the membrane in synaptosomes; additionally, it affects the architecture of proteins that act as receptors and channels. Several studies have studied the effects of DHA in SCI, with treatments that include intravenous bolus, nutritional supplementation, and the use of transgenic [47]. In SCI in rats, a single application of DHA (250 nmol/kg, i.v., 30 min after injury) showed an improvement in motor recovery, smaller lesion size, greater survival of neurons and oligodendrocytes, and lower oxidation of DNA/RNA in comparison to rats without treatment [48]. More details of the application of DHA in SCI are mentioned in the chapter on Samaddar [47], as well as interesting effects on molecules involved in the repair and conservation of axonal integrity.

3.5 Endogenous antioxidants (vitamins C, D, and E and ubiquinol)

Several molecules that already act as endogenous antioxidants have been studied as candidates for application in antioxidant therapies for SCI. Vitamin C, or ascorbic acid, is a small water-soluble molecule that has a double bond and participates in various metabolic processes as a reducing agent. It is considered nontoxic because it does not accumulate and its concentration declines during SCI. In rats, it decreases tissue inflammation and necrosis and only at high doses (200 mg/kg i.p. 1-h post-injury, daily, until they were sacrificed, 4th week) showed improvements in motor evaluations [49]. Vitamin D (1,25-dihydroxyvitamin D3, VDH, active form) is a molecule with cholesterol skeleton and acts similarly to hormones and steroids on several systems. Its receptor (VDR) is widely distributed in the CNS, and it apparently acts on the same targets as progesterone through similar pathways. Its use in CNS damage models in vivo and in vitro has shown promising results on several aspects. The prolongation or exacerbation of inflammation also gives way to greater damage by oxidative stress; therefore, the effect of VDH in vivo on the inhibition of iNOS and increase of IL-4 and TGF-β and in vitro modulating the production of molecules involved in oxidative stress, neurotoxic damage, and axonal growth on various cells are of interest for being use in SCI [50]. Tocopherols are a group of four fat-soluble phenolic compounds designated α, β, γ, and δ, which are found in vegetable oils, being alpha (α-T, considered the classic vitamin E) the one with the highest proportion in blood and tissues. All tocopherols are strong chain breaking antioxidants by effectively scavenging ROS and RNS. α-T significantly reduces the activity of iNOS and COX-2 [51]; in addition, the effect of extracts or synthetic derivatives has been evaluated, decreasing cell death due to excitotoxicity and oxidative stress in astrocytes [52] and accelerating remyelination of focal demyelinated lesions chemically induced [53]. In rats with SCI, the use of α-T (600 mg/kg i.m., twice weekly, for 6 weeks) decreased the damage caused by ischemia-reperfusion, improving the levels of motor and sensory recovery and the level of oxidative stress [54]. Ubiquinol (reduced form) or coenzyme Q10 is among the antioxidants that decrease their concentration after SCI. It is a fat-soluble cofactor present in the inner mitochondrial membrane acting as an antioxidant in the respiratory chain. Previously, the effect on ischemia-reperfusion damage in the CNS has been proven, preventing LP and reducing the size of the lesions [55].

3.6 Immunotherapy

The use of antibodies in the treatment of SCI is diverse and is directed to the functions of immune cells involved in inflammation and the pathological process. The initial invasion of leukocytes depends on the interaction of CD11d/CD18 (cluster of differentiation; CD) integrin with vascular cell adhesion molecule-1 (VCAM-1). In the case of the use of anti-CD11d monoclonal antibody administered in rats to determinate the therapeutic window with 1 mg/kg doses i.v. on groups at different times of application (2, 6, 12, 24, or 48 h post-lesion), it was shown that the treatment beginning even up to 6 h after the lesion resulted in an attenuation of infiltrating leukocytes (neutrophils and macrophages, sources of ROS and RNS), lowered the expression of COX-2 and iNOS, and lowered the amounts of HNE, NT-3, and dinitrophenyl (DNP) (used for the detection of protein carbonylation) therefore acting as an indirect antioxidant. This treatment also showed improvement in motor recovery vs. a control antibody [56]. Another important integrin is the dimer α4β1 also known as very late antigen 4 (VLA-4), and treatments with anti-α4 blocking monoclonal antibodies (2.5 mg/kg/2 and 24 h/i.v.) or small molecule blocker BIO5192 (10 mg/kg/2 h/continuous i.v. infusion for assessment of oxidative damage) showed a decreased influx of neutrophils/macrophages, reduced oxidant activity (COX-2, NO or iNOS, MDA), preserved white and gray matter, improved motor function in different evaluations, and decreased mechanical allodynia after SCI, when compared with the controls [57, 58].

3.7 Antioxidant peptides

3.7.1 A91 peptide

Modified neural peptides are peptide analogs of the myelin basic protein (MBP) epitopes that possess one or more aa substitutions and that have a partial agonist or antagonist action when in contact with the T lymphocyte (TL) receptor [59, 60].

Schwartz and Hauben tested the administration of non-encephalitogenic peptides of different aa sequences associated with MBP, which are named according to the position of the aa substitution that is performed: A96, G91, and A91, among others. A91 showed the best results after a traumatic injury, both in the optic nerve and in spinal cord, without showing clinical signs of autoimmune disease, hypersensitivity, immunosuppression, and controlling the destructive action of autoreactive TL [61, 62].

A91 is a peptide belonging to the aa 87–99 sequence of MBP with the substitution of an aa at position 91 of a lysine (VHFF<u>K</u>NIVTPRTP) by an alanine (VHFF<u>A</u>NIVTPRTP), functioning as a partial agonist peptide and promoting a change of the profile of cytokines produced by TL reactive against the 87–99 sequence of the MBP of a Th1 phenotype (interferon gamma [IFN-γ], TNF, IL-2) to a Th2 (IL-4, IL-10) and decreasing the action and synthesis of the FR, among other effects [63]. A91 allows activating the microglia with a phenotype producing neurotrophic factors, which together with the release of factors produced by other cells such as monocytes (MN) and TL reduce secondary neuronal degeneration [64–66].

The beneficial effect of subcutaneous immunization at the base of the tail has been demonstrated with A91 at a single dose (150–200 μg/kg) after SCI due to moderate contusion. This immunization, among various factors and effects, promotes neuroprotection and motor recovery by decreasing the expression of iNOS and production of $NO^{\bullet}$, LP, caspase 3, and pro-inflammatory cytokines and increasing the release of neurotrophic factors such as BDNF and NT-3. The effect of the immunization is preserved in the chronic stage of the lesion and as a prophylactic treatment or up to 72 h after the SCI; however, it diminishes when applied to lesions due to severe contusion or complete medullar cut and is eliminated with a double immunization. It has also been determined that the severity of the lesion determines the profile of genetic expression in the lesion after immunization and that immunization plus the removal of the fibroglial scar and/or the implant of a scaffold as support for mesenchymal stem cells favors a permissive microenvironment for motor recovery and improves the electrophysiological activity in the chronic stage after a complete section of the spinal cord [67–73]. The protective response of A91 is between 4 and 6 days, indicating that it acts on subsequent mechanisms to the acute stage. During this time, the oxidative processes are not completely modulated. Regarding this, it has been shown that the therapeutic combination of A91 peptide with peptides acting at shorter times, such as glutathione monoethyl ester (GSH-MEE) or the monocyte locomotion inhibitory factor (MLIF), reduces FR and LP and induces better motor recovery, neural survival, presence of myelinated axons, and tissue protection. In the same way, it was demonstrated that the combination of A91 with GSH-MEE retains the effect if applied until 72 hrs after the lesion [68, 74, 75].

3.7.2 Monocyte locomotion inhibitory factor (MLIF) peptide

MLIF is a pentapeptide (Met-Gln-Cys-Asn-Ser). In vitro studies showed that MLIF decreases MN locomotion, the production of ROS (H_2O_2, $O_2^{\bullet-}$, $HO^{\bullet}$), $NO^{\bullet}$, and cGMP, and it induces an increase of microtubules associated to the centriole and the concentration of cAMP [76–78]. The pharmacophore group of the MLIF is integrated by the Cys-Asn-Ser tripeptide, which retains the same biological activities of the factor [79, 80].

The MLIF favors the Th2 response; modulates the synthesis of pro-/anti-inflammatory cytokines and the expression of genes involved in inflammation, proliferation, angiogenesis, synthesis/degradation of extracellular matrix, angiogenesis, and axonal guidance, among others; and acts mainly through the signaling pathways: NF-kB, MAPKinases, and eEF1A1/endothelial nitric oxide synthase [81–84].

In vivo, the factor retards the arrival of MN in Rebuck windows and inhibits cutaneous delayed hypersensitivity to dinitrochlorobenzene, while in guinea pigs, it lobs down the expression of VLA-4 and VCAM-1 adhesion molecules in postcapillary vascular endothelium and decreases the formation of pericardial adhesions in rats when applied directly to the site of injury after surgery [85].

Studies in cerebral ischemia showed that the penetrating, antioxidant, anti-inflammatory, and neuroprotective capacity of the pharmacophore group is favored in analogs when the N-terminal end is modified by adding one of the following aa: Asp, His, Try, or Arg. In the same way, cardioprotective effects have been seen in myocardial ischemia [86, 87]. On the other hand, pharmacokinetic studies are underway to determine the concentration of MLIF in plasma [88].

In base studies of our group, rats were subjected to a moderate SCI, and a dose of 200 μg of MLIF was applied directly to the site of the lesion. The animals treated with the factor presented a greater motor recovery than the non-treated, and a decrease in the LP, the concentration of $NO^{\bullet}$, and the expression of the iNOS. An increase in the expression of the IL-10 and TGF-β (Transforming Growth Factor beta) genes was observed at 3 h and 7 days post-injury, favoring the survival of the ventral horn neurons [75]. Subsequent studies showed that four doses of the MLIF at the same concentration immediately initiating direct administration at the site of injury and subsequently one dose every 24 h for 3 days by i.p. administration are sufficient to improve motor recovery in rats subjected to SCI. In the same way, therapeutic combinations of MLIF, at different times and doses, have favored the effect of the MLIF in the experimental model of SCI modulating the synthesis of the FR and ROS.

3.7.3 Glutathione (GSH) peptide

GSH (**Figure 3**) is a tripeptide (L-γ-glutamyl-L-cysteinyl-glycine), nonprotein thiol. It is synthesized in the cellular cytoplasm by the consecutive action of two enzymes. The first, γ-glutamylcysteinyl ligase, is regulated by the nuclear factor (erythroid-derived 2)-like 2 (NFE2L2 or Nrf2), which is sensitive to oxidative stress. This enzyme uses glutamic acid (Glu) and Cys aa, glutamic acid (Glu) and Cys aa, as a substrate to form the γ-glutamylcysteine dipeptide (γ-GluCys), which

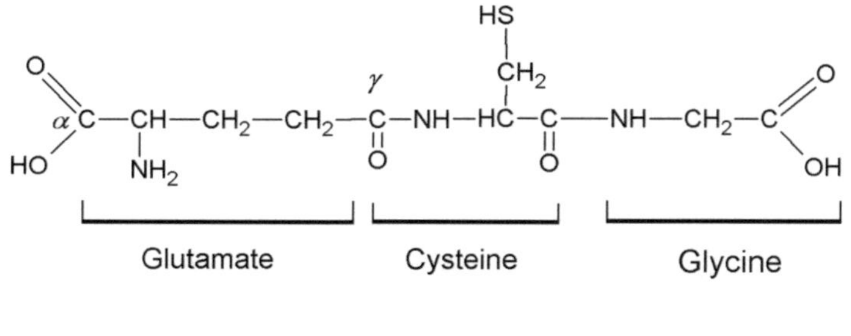

Figure 3.
Condensed structural chemical formula of glutathione (IUPAC name: (2S)-2-amino-4-{[(1R)-1-[(carboxymethyl) carbomoyl]-2-sulfanylethyl] carbomyl1} butanoic acid). Modified from Gaucher et al. [89].

is combined with glycine (Gly) in a reaction catalyzed by the second enzyme (glutathione synthase) to form GSH, whose concentration is regulated by the nhibition of γ-GluCys ligase, the cellular content of L-cysteine, and the final concentration of GSH. Thus, the intracellular and extracellular concentrations of GSH are determined by the balance among its synthesis, catabolism, and transport between cytosol and the different organelles [89].

GSH, by itself, is not transported effectively into the cells, and under normal physiological conditions, it is in a reduced form. During its oxidation (where the thiol group of Cys is responsible for the redox reactions) by ROS and RNS, it involves two types of reactions, a nonenzymatic reaction with the $NO^{\bullet}$, HO^{-}, and $O_2^{\bullet -}$ radicals and an enzymatic one providing an electron for the reduction of peroxides in the reaction, catalyzed by GPx to form the oxidized glutathione GSSG (two GSH molecules bound by the disulfide bridge), which is regenerated by Gr, an enzyme that transfers electrons from NADPH to GSSG by reducing it [90, 91]. Thus, the redox state of GSH activates the activator protein 1 (AP-1) responsible for the expression of cytokine genes, TGF-β, and collagenase and AP-2 responsible for the activation of c-Jun-N-terminal kinases (JNK), stress-activated protein kinases (SAPK), protein kinase c (PK-C), and tyrosine kinase, while the decrease in the GSH level stimulates the activation of NF-κB, protein kinase B, c-Jun N-terminal Kinase, and mitogen-activated protein kinase with the subsequent increase in synthesis of pro-inflammatory cytokines and caspases. In suitable concentrations, GSH increases the activation, proliferation, and cellular differentiation and regulates the Ca^{2+} homeostasis [91], granting a fundamental role in cellular homeostasis and pathologies related to patient's age and oxidative stress states, such as neurodegenerative, neuroinflammatory, cardiovascular diseases, and cerebral ischemia, among others [92, 93]. To increase the intracellular GSH concentration levels, GSH precursors have been used, without modifying the Cys that is critical for the functioning of the peptide. GSH precursor molecules such as N-acetyl cysteine (NAC) stimulate the biosynthesis of GSH that acts directly on ROS, RNS [89, 93, 94], and glutathione esters, mainly mono- and dimethyl esters such as glutathione monoethyl ester [γ- Glu-Cys-Gly-OEt (GSH-MEE)], where the carboxyl group of Gly is esterified and, due to its high hydrophobicity, increases its permeability to the cell membrane and facilitates its transport in brain-spinal fluid [95–97]. Once GSH-MEE is located in the cellular cytoplasm, it is hydrolyzed by the intracellular esterases to release and cause the intracellular increase in the GSH concentration and react with the FR without enzymatic intervention or it reduces the peroxides by means of GPx through its oxidation to GSSG [89, 91, 98, 99].

GSH-MEE has been used effectively to protect cells from oxidizing agents and various toxic compounds in various cell lines and animal models with neurodegenerative and inflammatory processes [92, 99, 100]. Studies of our group and collaborators have shown that the i.p. administration of 12 mg/kg of GSH-MEE divided into four doses in the first 24 h post-lesion in rats subjected to a moderate SCI contributes to the reduction of oxidative stress, significantly improves motor function and survival of red core neurons, and stabilizes spinal cord blood flow [100], while a therapeutic combination of GSH-MEE (at the same dose and under the same scheme) with intradermal application (i.d.) of the A91 peptide at the base of the tail at a dose of 600 μg/kg immediately after the injury promotes a better neurological recovery and morphological preservation. This combination is able to maintain its neuroprotective action even if it starts 72 h after the injury [68, 74]. In the same way, our group has demonstrated that the therapeutic combination of GSH-MEE and MLIF promotes greater motor recovery and maintains several morphological aspects on the site of lesion in rats subjected to moderate SCI.

3.8 Natural extracts as antioxidants

A variety of ingredients and active ingredients derived from herbal extracts, known for their antioxidant and anti-inflammatory activity, have also called the attention to complement SCI treatments. Among all these, ingredients such as curcumin, resveratrol, epigallocatechin gallate, ligustrazine, quercitrin, and puerarin and herbs such as Dashen, *Ginkgo biloba*, Ginseng, Notoginseng, and Astragali Radix are outlined as candidates for various experimental studies. In the review by Zhang et al. [101], the molecular structures, application, and dose are listed, as well as the results found at a molecular level on SCI. In particular, the compound curcumin is a polyphenol substance isolated from the yellow extract from rhizome of *Curcuma longa*, and it has been widely used for medicinal purposes due to its potent effect in inhibiting acute and chronic inflammation. Regarding its antioxidant action, its application in SCI (300 mg/kg in DMSO, single dose i.p. after injury) has shown a decrease in MDA and an increase in SOD at 24 h [102], and at a lower dose, it has also increased the concentration and induction of GSH, GPx, and Nrf2 and decreased the expression of NF-κB, TNF-α, and IL-1β [101].

3.9 Spin trappings

A highly studied antioxidant strategy consists of scavengers of FR that include, among others, thiols (lipoic acid), GSH precursors, NAC, polyphenolic compounds, hydroxyl stilbenes, nitrones, and spin trappings (noncyclic and cyclic nitrones); we will only review the latter. Most spin trappings have a nitronate or nitroxide nucleus and are chemical agents that react with FR, forming stable products (adducts), and were originally developed as a tool to detect and stabilize the FR in chemistry and later in biological oxidation processes [103–105]. The first spin trappings had short half-lives and generated toxic $HO^{\bullet}$. By designing the spin trappings with the inclusion of heterocyclic rings (pyrrolines or phenol, generating Imidazolyl-nitrones, Furil-nitrones, Arylnitrons, and others) toxicity was reduced, improving its neuroprotective, anti-inflammatory, functionality, stability, bioavailability, and trapping different types of FR centered on O_2, carbon, and sulfur derivatives. In turn, this increases their solubility in high concentrations in a large number of solvents (~0.1M), producing a positive effect when administered in a varied-dose scheme before or after a traumatic event [103, 106]. A basic example of the nitrones is phenyl N-tert-butylnitrone (PBN), an arylnitrone with general formula X-CN = NO-Y, which acts by reacting with $O_2^{\bullet-}$ and/or HO^- to produce adducts. Once the adduct is formed, the radical is inactivated and unable to damage the cell tissue [104, 107]. The general reaction is that of the formation of adduct, schematized in **Figure 4**. In general, it is indicated that PBN is not toxic and the suitable concentration to form adducts is 10–15 mg/100 g of weight, while the estimated lethal dose is 10 times higher (100–150 mg/100 g of weight) [108]. The first neuroprotective evidence was in neurodegenerative models administered at low doses after injury and in the

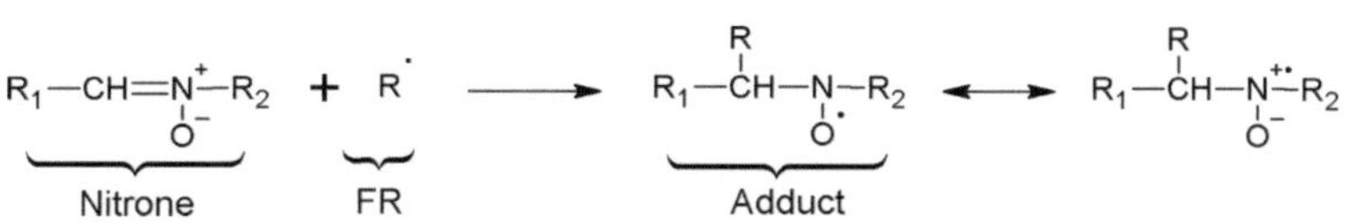

Figure 4.
Basic reaction of a nitrone with FR to produce a stable spin product (adduct). Modified from Refs. [105, 106].

prevention of stroke-induced mortality in models of ischemia in gerbils [103, 104, 109–113]. The pharmacological effects of PBN in animal models are extensive, protecting against death after endotoxic shock, bacterial meningitis, teratogenicity induced by thalidomide, diabetogenesis, hepatocarcinogenesis, etc. Many studies have reported a neuroprotective effect in SCI and the brain (the most studied) decreasing the expression of genes associated with apoptosis, inflammation, and iNOS by decreasing the activation of MAP p-38 NF-κB nitrogen kinase and synthesis of $NO^{\bullet}$ [114]. In a process of ischemia or perfusion, PBN reduces the size of the infarct by increasing ischemic reperfusion and decreasing neurodegeneration, excitotoxicity, and the activation of microglia; it also induces neurite growth through indirect activation of the Ras-ERK pathway, increasing animal survival [106, 115–117]. The neuroprotective effect of PBN is attributed to its ability to quickly and easily penetrate the membranes and the blood-brain barrier with a half-life of 3 h in plasma; decrease the levels of oxidized proteins, 8-isoprostane, HNE, IL-1β, TNF-α, IFN-γ, c-fos, IL-3, IL-4, IL-5, and H_2O_2; and favor an increase of GHS and IL-10, among others [106, 117–119]. In a model of cortical contusion in rats, it was demonstrated that pre-treatment with PBN with a single intravenous dose of 30 mg/kg 30 min before the injury reduces the cognitive deficit and its volume; it has shown to have a wide therapeutic window in focal ischemia rodent models, reducing the infarct volume when administered up to 12 h after the beginning of the stroke and reducing the loss of tissue when administered by fluid percussion 30 min. After injury in rats [120]. Currently, the nitrones derived from PBN [102] are being widely studied as neuroprotective in different CNS pathologies and in traumatic lesions. For example, 2,4-disulfophenyl-N-tert-butylnitrone (NXY-059) has neuroprotective effects when applied 4–5 hr post-occlusion at equimolar doses to PBN and reduced infarct volume from 37.2 to 12.5% when 30 mg/kg was administered i.v. 1 h after reperfusion in Wistar rats [121–124]. Meanwhile, stilbazulenyl nitrone (STAZN) exerts similar effects at lower doses than the one used for NXY-059; in fact, the tolerability and safety of NXY-059 were studied in patients with acute stroke in clinical trials [103, 124]. Although not all compounds have demonstrated their neuroprotective effect when administered 24 h after the traumatic event, some of them have allowed favoring the therapeutic window at repeated doses [103].

Other derivatives are 5,5-dimethyl-1-pyrroline-N-oxide (DMPO) and diesterified nitrone (EMEPO), which have shown similarities to the action of PBN but with some other advantages, such as being less toxic and increasing the levels of antiapoptotic proteins such as Bcl2 and p-Bad and decreasing the synthesis of pro-apoptotic ones such as caspase 3, p53, and Bax [125–127]. In addition, (2, 2, 6, 6-tetramethylpiperidin-1-yl)oxyl (Tempo) and (4-hydroxy-2,2,6,6-tetramethylpiperidin-1-yl)oxyl (Tempol) have shown antioxidant properties in radiation damage and injury [128, 129]. In a traumatic brain injury mouse model, Tempol reduced post-traumatic LP and oxidative damage induced by protein nitration, decreasing mitochondrial damage, cytoskeletal damage, and neurodegeneration and improving motor function [128, 130, 131].

Despite the results observed with the nitrones and the wide range of studies performed for therapeutic uses at different doses and times, their action is attributed to their ability to form adducts, but not before indicating the possible participation of other mechanisms that favor their neuroprotective activity, thus expanding the information on antioxidant therapy strategies in the clinical area.

3.10 Polyethylene glycol (PEG)-superoxide dismutase (SOD)

Polyethylene glycol (PEG) is a surfactant that due to its hydrophilic nature allows the fusion and fluidity of the cell membrane that reduces the oxidative effects of the secondary stage and that during the acute phase of SCI, it may inhibit nerve fiber degeneration and create a favorable microenvironment for the regeneration of nerve filaments that can stimulate angiogenesis and reduce glial scar, promoting the regeneration of axonal guidance and motor recovery. PEG has been widely used as a scaffold for a large variety of molecules in treatment for SCI [132–136], while the SOD enzyme has antioxidant properties, as mentioned previously. The combination of SOD with PEG (PEG-SOD) allows an increase of the enzyme intracellularly and its antioxidant activity, and it may have an important role in vascular relaxation by reducing the concentration of $O2^{\bullet -}$ and limiting the LP [132]. It has been used in myocardial ischemia and in lung injury models, proposed as a treatment vs. oxidative stress [132].

In a controlled phase II study in patients in a coma who suffered a stroke and received a single i.v. dose of 2000, 5000, or 10,000 IU/kg 4 h after the injury, its recovery was better in comparison to the group that received placebo (44% were in a vegetative state or died); no side effects were observed in this study due to the administration of the drug [137].

In a study in a cerebral ischemia model performed in rats, 10,000 IU/kg of PSG-SOD were i.v. administered, and the group presented a significant reduction in infarct size in comparison to the control group [138]. In other study with Sprague-Dawley male rats (300-350g of weight), an occlusion of the hepatic artery was performed and reperfusion was performed after 90 min to generate liver damage. A group of animals received i.v. 5000 U/kg of PEG-SOD before vascular occlusion and immediately after reperfusion, while the control group only received a saline solution following the same scheme. In the group treated with PEG-SOD, hepatic ischemia and LP were attenuated. Meanwhile, another study examined the effect of PEG-SOD on focal cerebral ischemia/reperfusion in rats; the results showed that the effect is variable, depending on the dosage [132, 139]. In a dog experiment, thoracic aortic cross-clamping was performed; a dose of 5000 U/kg of PEG-SOD was i.v. administered to one group 15–20 min before clamping, and the other group only received a saline solution. Delayed paraplegia was avoided in the group of dogs that received the conjugate, unlike the groups that did not receive it [140]. Edward et al. conducted an important review of the use of PEG-SOD in phase II and III studies in traumatic brain injury [141].

3.11 Mannitol

When mannitol is used for medical purposes, it is administered intravenously. Mannitol can be found in varying concentrations, dissolved in 100 mL of fluid (5, 20, and 25% mannitol). A common solution is 20% mannitol. Cruz and colleagues described the dose-response effect of preoperative mannitol on acute subdural hematomas in traumatic brain injury in which mannitol therapy has been classically directed, establishing and maintaining an osmotic gradient between the blood and brain [142, 143].

Maintaining an adequate spinal cord perfusion pressure is crucial after SCI. Intramedullary edema within the spinal cord and consecutively raised intrathecal pressure at the injury are important secondary injury mechanisms in the pathobiology after traumatic SCI. Increased intraspinal pressure reduces spinal cord perfusion pressure, which leads to worsen post-traumatic ischemia [144].

Mannitol allows the control of blood flow patterns in the spinal cord; it has been used experimentally in some studies in rats that have suffered a controlled SCI and in dogs/cats that suffer an SCI within the clinical area. Mannitol is recommended to reduce the effect of inflammation and edema, an effect that has been corroborated with microangiographic and electrophysiological studies. One hour after the application of a 3 g/kg dose, an improved intramedullary vascular pattern was detected among the animals treated with mannitol compared to those that were not treated, and 4 h after the perfusion, many areas of the lateral white matter of the spinal cord were almost normal [145]. In a study in dogs, an SCI was experimentally induced, and it was reported that mannitol alone did not help to reverse the paralysis of these animals [146]; however, another study stated that the i.v. administration of mannitol at a dose of 2 g/kg had a good effect on the white matter of the spinal cord and areas of the brain [147]. In a retrospective study with Sprague-Dawley rats, a group with SCI by compression by means of a clamp, 2 g/kg mannitol were administered immediately after the injury, while the control group was given 0.9% saline solution; all groups underwent structural and electrophysiological studies. The group treated with mannitol obtained excellent results, finding significant improvement in neural structures and protection of the spinal cord after SCI [148]. In a study in dogs to which an edema was induced by severe external spinal cord trauma, 3 g/kg of mannitol was i.v. administered, and they were neurologically evaluated, and a myelography study was performed after 2 h of the treatment, to identify the edema, showing that there was reduction of it [149].

3.12 Combinatory therapies and results in symptoms of SCI

In addition to its independent use, several studies have evaluated the use of one or more antioxidants together by themselves or in addition to other existing therapies for SCI, such as rehabilitation exercise or cell transplantation, expecting a synergism to enhance the recovery. Moreover, some therapies not only aim to improve the immediate treatment of SCI but also improve the effects it has on relieving the most common complications in patients. To mention some, the combination of vitamin C as antioxidant (100 mg/kg/1 h and daily/28d, i.p.) together with the transplantation of bone marrow mesenchymal stem cells (BMMSC) (3×10^6 cells) induced improvements in motor recovery in rats when compared with methylprednisolone (MP), vitamin C, or BMMSC alone in SCI [150]; simultaneous administration of vitamin D (5 μg/kg/twice daily) and progesterone (0.5 mg/kg/twice daily i.m.) for 5 days demonstrated a higher efficacy in reducing neuroinflammation in comparison to when they were administered separately, and when they were administrated early (first 4 h) in SCI patients receiving MP, there was improvement in the motor and sensory functions 6 months after starting therapy [151]. Applying once a day a combination of low-dose fluoxetine (1 mg/kg/i.p.) and vitamin C (100 mg/kg/i.p.) immediately after the event and for 14 days had a protective effect on the BSCB integrity, improving the functional recovery, showing inhibition of the expression and activation of the matrix metalloproteinase, and decreasing the infiltration of leukocytes and the expression of inflammatory and oxidizing molecules, but not when they were applied separately in rats [152]. In SCI patients, dietary supplementation for 3 months, which included three 750 mg per day of omega-3 fatty acids and antioxidants (400 mg of mixed tocopherols, coenzyme Q10, curcumin, etc.), caused a decrease of inflammatory cytokines with reduction in neuropathic pain [153]; 2 months vitamin E dietary supplementation 765–1020 IU/day in rats before SCI showed accelerated bladder recovery, significant motor improvement, and a high number of oligodendrocytes compared to the controls [154].

4. Conclusion

After a primary injury occurs on the spinal cord, destructive biochemical mechanisms are initiated (secondary injury) that play a fundamental role in the pathophysiology of spinal cord injury. Within these, oxidative stress and lipid peroxidation exacerbate the biochemical mechanisms once initiated and propagate neurodegenerative damage, so the degree of loss of long-term motor and sensory functions depends largely on their intensity. This damage suffered during the acute phase and that may be irreversible requires a timely intervention. To guarantee the antioxidant effect that will render better results, it is important to consider the new agents and therapies in the SCI treatment at the appropriate times. There is no fully restorative therapy for SCI, but strategies for the modulation of this damage contribute to neuroprotection and, although partially, to functional recovery.

Acknowledgements

We are grateful for the support given to the line of research related to the evaluation of immunomodulatory peptides in oxidative stress under the support No. FIS/IMSS/PROT/G16/1605 and FIS /IMSS/PROT/G17/1676 and the scholarship granted to the students of Master's degree Dulce M. Parra and Jonathan Vilchis by CONACYT and IMSS.

Conflict of interest

The authors declare no competing financial interests.

Acronyms and abbreviations

aa	amino acids
ADH	alcohol dehydrogenase
ALDH	aldehyde dehydrogenase
BSCB	blood-spinal cord barrier
BMMSC	bone marrow mesenchymal stem cells
CAT	catalase
CD	cluster of differentiation
CNS	central nervous system
$CO_3^{\bullet-}$	carbonate radical
COX	cyclooxygenase
DHA	docosahexaenoic acid
DNP	dinitrophenyl
EPA	eicosapentaenoic acid
ER	estrogen receptor
FR	free radicals
GAP-43	growth-associated protein 43
GFAP	glial fibrillary acidic protein
GPx	glutathione peroxidases
GR	glutathione reductases
GSH	glutathione, reduced
GSH-MEE	glutathione monoethyl ester
GSSG	glutathione, oxidized
GST	glutathione S-transferases
HNE	4-hydroxy-2-nonenal
H_2O_2	hydrogen peroxide
$HO^{\bullet}$	hydroxyl radical
HO^-	hydroxyl anion

IFN-γ	interferon gamma
IL	interleukin
iNOS	inducible nitric synthase
$L^{\bullet}$	lipid radical
LH	lipid
LP	lipid peroxidation
$LOO^{\bullet}$	lipid peroxyl radical
$LO^{\bullet}$	lipid alkoxyl radical
LOOH	lipid hydroperoxide
MLIF	monocyte locomotion inhibitory factor
MDA	malondialdehyde
MP or MPSS	methylprednisolone sodium succinate
NAC	N-acetyl cysteine
NADPH	nicotinamide-adenine dinucleotide phosphate, reduced
$NO^{\bullet}$	nitric oxide
$NO_2^{\bullet -}$	nitrogen dioxide radical
NOS	nitric oxide synthase
NT-3	3-nitrotyrosine
$O_2^{\bullet -}$	superoxide
$OONO^-$	peroxynitrite
PBN	phenyl N-tert-butylnitrone
PEG	polyethylene glycol
PEG-SOD	polyethylene glycol-superoxide dismutase
PUFA	polyunsaturated fatty acid
ROS	reactive oxygen species
RNS	reactive nitrogen species
$RO_2^{\bullet}/HO_2^{\bullet}$	peroxyl radical
SCI	spinal cord injury
SOD	superoxide dismutase
TGF-β	transforming growth factor beta
TNF-α	tumor necrosis factor alpha
VCAM-1	vascular cell adhesion molecule-1
VDH	vitamin D: 1,25-dihydroxyvitamin D3
VLA-4	very late antigen 4
XO	xanthine oxidase

Author details

Jonathan Vilchis Villa, Dulce M. Parra Villamar, José Alberto Toscano Zapien, Liliana Blancas Espinoza, Juan Herrera García and Raúl Silva García*
Medical Research Unit in Immunology, Hospital of Pediatric "Dr. Silvestre Frenk Freund"—CMN, SXXI, IMSS, Mexico City, Mexico

*Address all correspondence to: silgarrul@yahoo.com.mx

References

[1] Fehlings MG, Wilson JR, Harrop JS. Efficacy and safety of methylprednisolone sodium succinate in acute spinal cord injury: A systematic review. Global Spine Journal. 2017;**7**(3S):116S-137S. DOI: 10.1177/2192568217706366

[2] Hall E, Wang JA, Bosken JM, et al. Lipid peroxidation in brain or spinal cord mitochondria after injury. Journal of Bioenergetics and Biomembranes. 2016;**48**(2):169-174. DOI: 10.1007/s10863-015-9600-5

[3] Oyimbo C. Secondary injury mechanisms in traumatic spinal cord injury: A nugget of this multiply cascade. Acta Neurobiologiae Experimentalis. 2011;**71**:281-299

[4] Pisoschi A, Pop A. The role of antioxidants in the chemistry of oxidative stress: A review. European Journal of Medicinal Chemistry. 2015;**97**:55-74. DOI: 10.1016/j.ejmech.2015.04.040

[5] Hall E. Antioxidant therapies for acute spinal cord injury. Neurotherapeutics. 2011;**8**(2):152-167. DOI: 10.1007/s13311-011-0026-4

[6] Gutteridge J. Biological origin of free radicals, and mechanisms of antioxidant protection. Chemico-Biological Interactions. 1994;**9**:133-140

[7] Kohen R, Ayska A. Oxidation of biological systems: Oxidative stress phenomena, antioxidants, redox reactions, and methods for their quantification. Toxicologic Pathology. 2002;**30**(6):620-650. DOI: 10.1080/01926230290166724

[8] Carballal S, Bartesaghi S, Radi R. Kinetic and mechanistic considerations to assess the biological fate of peroxynitrite. Biochimica et Biophysica Acta. 2014;**1840**(2):768-780. DOI: 10.1016/j.bbagen.2013.07.005

[9] Anthonymuthu T, Kenny EM, Bayir H. Therapies targeting lipid peroxidation in traumatic brain injury. Brain Research. 2016;**1640**(1 Pt A):57-76. DOI: 10.1016/j.brainres.2016.02.006

[10] Salem N, Lin M, Moriguchi Y, et al. Distribution of omega-6 and omega-3 polyunsaturated fatty acids in the whole rat body and 25 compartments. Prostaglandins, Leukotrienes, and Essential Fatty Acids. 2015;**100**:13-20. DOI: 10.1016/j.plefa.2015.06.002

[11] Lushchak V. Free radicals, reactive oxygen species, oxidative stress and its classification. Chemico-Biological Interactions. 2014;**224**:164-175. DOI: 10.1016/j.cbi.2014.10.016

[12] Gaschler MM, Stockwell BR. Lipid peroxidation in cell death. Biochemical and Biophysical Research Communications. 2017;**482**(3):419-425. DOI: 10.1016/j.bbrc.2016.10.086

[13] Spickett C. The lipid peroxidation product 4-hydroxy-2-nonenal: Advances in chemistry and analysis. Redox Biology. 2013;**1**:145-152. DOI: 10.1016/j.redox.2013.01.007

[14] Singhal S, Singh S, Singhal P, et al. Antioxidant role of glutathione S-Transferases: 4-Hydroxynonenal, a key molecule in stress-mediated Signaling. Toxicology and Applied Pharmacology. 2015;**289**(3):361-370. DOI: 10.1016/j.taap.2015.10.006

[15] Ji Y, Dai Z, Wu G, et al. 4-Hydroxy-2-nonenal induces apoptosis by activating ERK1/2 signaling and depleting intracellular glutathione in intestinal epithelial cells. Scientific Reports. 2016;**6**:32929. DOI: 10.1038/srep32929

[16] Ayala A, Muñoz MF, Argüelles S. Lipid peroxidation: production, metabolism, and signaling

mechanisms of malondialdehyde and 4-hydroxy-2-nonenal. Oxidative Medicine and Cellular Longevity. 2014;**2014**:31. Article ID 360438. DOI: 10.1155/2014/360438

[17] Stadtman E, Levine R. Free radical-mediated oxidation of free amino acids and amino acid residues in proteins. Amino Acids. 2003;**25**:207-218. DOI: 10.1007/s00726-003-0011-2

[18] Møller I, Rogowska W, Rao R. Protein carbonylation and metal-catalysed protein oxidation in a cellular perspective. Journal of Proteomics. 2011;**74**(11):2228-2242. doi.org.conricyt.remotexs.co. DOI: 10.1016/j.jprot.2011.05.004

[19] Castro J, Jung T, Grune T, Siems W. 4-Hydroxynonenal (HNE) modified proteins in metabolic diseases. Free Radical Biology and Medicine. 2017;**11**:309-315. DOI: 10.1016/j.freeradbiomed.2016.10.497

[20] Zarkovic N, Cipak A, Jaganjac M, et al. Pathophysiological relevance of aldehydic protein modifications. Journal of Proteomics. 2013;**92**:239-247. DOI: 10.1016/j.jprot.2013.02.004

[21] Lubieniecka J, Streijger F, Lee J, et al. Biomarkers for severity of spinal cord injury in the cerebrospinal fluid of rats. PLoS One. 2011;**6**(4):e19247. DOI: 10.1371/journal.pone.0019247

[22] Hulme C, Brown H, Fuller S, et al. The developing landscape of diagnostic and prognostic biomarkers for spinal cord injury in cerebrospinal fluid and blood. Spinal Cord. 2017;**55**:114-125. DOI: 10.1038/sc.2016.174

[23] Niedzielska E, Irena Smaga I, Gawlik M, et al. Oxidative stress in neurodegenerative diseases. Molecular Neurobiology. 2016;**53**:4094-4125. DOI: 10.1007/s12035-015-9337-5

[24] Dalleau S, Baradat M, Gueraud F, et al. Cell death and diseases related to oxidative stress: 4-hydroxynonenal (HNE) in the balance. Cell Death and Differentiation. 2013;**20**(12):1615-1630. DOI: 10.1038/cdd.2013.138

[25] Huang H, Kozekov I, Kozekova A, et al. DNA crosslink induced by trans-4-hydroxynonenal. Environmental and Molecular Mutagenesis. 2010;**51**(6):625-634. DOI: 10.1002/em.20599

[26] Minko I, Kozekov I, Harris T, et al. Chemistry and biology of DNA containing 1,N2-deoxyguanosine adducts of the α,β-unsaturated aldehydes acrolein, crotonaldehyde, and 4-hydroxynonenal. Chemical Research in Toxicology. 2009;**22**(5):759-778. DOI: 10.1021/tx9000489

[27] Bains B, Hall ED. Antioxidant therapies in traumatic brain and spinal cord injury. Biochimica et Biophysica Acta. 2012;**1822**(5):675-684. DOI: 10.1016/j.bbadis.2011.10.017

[28] Mol M, Regazzoni L, Altomare A, et al. Enzymatic and non-enzymatic detoxification of 4-hydroxynonenal: Methodological aspects and biological consequences. Free Radical Biology and Medicine. 2017;**111**:328-344. DOI: 10.1016/j.freeradbiomed.2017.01.036

[29] Zhang H, Squadrito G, Uppu R, et al. Pryor reaction of peroxynitrite with melatonin: A mechanistic study. Chemical Research in Toxicology. 1999;**12**(6):526-534. DOI: 10.1021/tx980243t

[30] Yang L, Yao M, Lan Y, et al. Melatonin for spinal cord injury in animal models: A systematic review and network meta-analysis. Journal of Neurotrauma. 2016;**33**(3):290-300. DOI: 10.1089/neu.2015.4038

[31] Shen Z, Zhou Z, Gao S, et al. Melatonin inhibits neural cell apoptosis and promotes locomotor recovery via activation of the Wnt/beta-catenin signaling pathway after spinal cord

injury. Neurochemical Research. 2017;**42**(8):2336-2343. DOI: 10.1007/s11064-017-2251-7

[32] Park S, Lee S, Park K, et al. Beneficial effects of endogenous and exogenous melatonin on neural reconstruction and functional recovery in an animal model of spinal cord injury. Journal of Pineal Research. 2012;**52**(1):107-119. DOI: 10.1111/j.1600-079X.2011.00925.x

[33] Jing Y, Wu Q, Yuan X, et al. Microvascular protective role of pericytes in melatonin-treated spinal cord injury in the C57BL/6 mice. Chinese Medical Journal (Engl). 2014;**127**(15):2808-2813

[34] Wu Q, Jing Y, Yuan X, et al. Melatonin treatment protects against acute spinal cord injury-induced disruption of blood spinal cord barrier in mice. Journal of Molecular Neuroscience. 2014;**54**(4):714-722. DOI: 10.1007/s12031-014-0430-4

[35] Aydemir S, Dogan D, Kocak A, et al. The effect of melatonin on spinal cord after ischemia in rats. Spinal Cord. 2016;**54**(5):360-363. DOI: 10.1038/sc.2015.204

[36] Genovese T, Mazzon E, Crisafulli C, et al. Effects of combination of melatonin and dexamethasone on secondary injury in an experimental mice model of spinal cord trauma. Journal of Pineal Research. 2007;**43**(2):140-153. DOI: 10.1111/j.1600-079X.2007.00454.x

[37] Longoni B, Salgo M, Pryor W, Marchiafava PL. Effects of melatonin on lipid peroxidation induced by oxygen radicals. Life Sciences. 1998;**62**(10):853-859

[38] Cayli S, Kocak A, Yilmaz U, et al. Effect of combined treatment with melatonin and methylprednisolone on neurological recovery after experimental spinal cord injury. European Spine Journal. 2004;**13**(8):724-732. DOI: 10.1007/s00586-003-0550-y

[39] Kalkan E, Cicek O, Unlu A, et al. The effects of prophylactic zinc and melatonin application on experimental spinal cord ischemia-reperfusion injury in rabbits: Experimental study. Spinal Cord. 2007;**45**(11):722-730. DOI: 10.1038/sj.sc.3102035

[40] Shultz RB, Zhong Y. Minocycline targets multiple secondary injury mechanisms in traumatic spinal cord injury. Neural Regeneration Research. 2017;**12**(5):702-713. DOI: 10.4103/1673-5374.206633

[41] Aras M, Altas M, Motor S, et al. Protective effects of minocycline on experimental spinal cord injury in rats. Injury-International Journal of the Care of the Injured. 2015;**46**:1471-1474. DOI: 10.1016/j.injury.2015.05.018

[42] Plane JM, Shen Y, Pleasure DE, et al. Prospects for minocycline neuroprotection. Archives of Neurology. 2010;**67**(12):1442-1448. DOI: 10.1001/archneurol.2010.191

[43] Casha S, Zygun D, McGowan MD, et al. Results of a phase II placebo-controlled randomized trial of minocycline in acute spinal cord injury. Brain. 2012;**135**(4):1224-1236. DOI: 10.1093/brain/aws072

[44] Chakrabarti M, Das A, Samantaray S, et al. Molecular mechanisms of estrogen for neuroprotection in spinal cord injury and traumatic brain injury. Reviews in the Neurosciences. 2016;**27**(3):271-281. DOI: 10.1515/revneuro-2015-0032

[45] Samantaray S, Das A, Banik NL, et al. Administration of low dose-estrogen attenuates persistent inflammation, promotes angiogenesis and improves locomotor function following chronic spinal cord injury in rats. Journal of

Neurochemistry. 2016;**137**(4):604-617. DOI: 10.1111/jnc.13610

[46] Colón JM, Torrado AI, Cajigas A, et al. Tamoxifen administration immediately or 24 hours after spinal cord injury improves Locomotor recovery and reduces secondary damage in female rats. Journal of Neurotrauma. 2016;**33**(18):1696-1708. DOI: 10.1089/neu.2015.4111

[47] Samaddar S. Effect of docosahexaenoic acid (DHA) on spinal cord injury. In: Essa M, Akbar M, Guillemin G, editors. The Benefits of Natural Products for Neurodegenerative Diseases, Advances in Neurobiology. Vol. 12. Cham: Springer; 2016. DOI: 10.1007/978-3-319-28383-8_2

[48] King VR, Huang WL, et al. Omega-3 fatty acids improve recovery, whereas omega-6 fatty acids worsen outcome, after spinal cord injury in the adult rat. The Journal of Neuroscience. 2006;**26**(17):4672-4680. DOI: 10.1523/JNEUROSCI.5539-05.2006

[49] Yan M, Yang M, Shao W, et al. High-dose ascorbic acid administration improves functional recovery in rats with spinal cord contusion injury. Spinal Cord. 2014;**52**(11):803-808. DOI: 10.1038/sc.2014.135

[50] Cekic M, Sayeed I, Stein DG. Combination treatment with progesterone and vitamin D hormone may Be more effective than monotherapy for nervous system injury and disease. Frontiers in Neuroendocrinology. 2009;**30**(2):158-172. DOI: 10.1016/j.yfrne.2009.04.002

[51] Devaraj S, Tang R, Adams-Huet B, et al. Effect of high-dose alpha-tocopherol supplementation on biomarkers of oxidative stress and inflammation and carotid atherosclerosis in patients with coronary artery disease. The American Journal of Clinical Nutrition. 2007;**86**:1392-1398. DOI: 10.1093/ajcn/86.5.1392

[52] Selvaraju TR, Khaza'ai H, Vidyadaran S, Abd Mutalib MS, Vasudevan R. The neuroprotective effects of tocotrienol rich fraction and alpha tocopherol against glutamate injury in astrocytes. Bosnian Journal of Basic Medical Sciences. 2014;**14**(4):195-204. DOI: 10.17305/bjbms.2014.4.91

[53] Blanchard B, Heurtaux T, García C, et al. Tocopherol derivative TFA-12 promotes myelin repair in experimental models of multiple sclerosis. The Journal of Neuroscience. 2013;**33**(28):11633-11642. DOI: 10.1523/JNEUROSCI.0774-13.2013

[54] Morsy MD, Mostaffa OA, Hassan WN. A potential protective effect of α-tocopherol on vascular complication in spinal cord reperfusion injury in rats. Journal of Biomedical Science. 2010;**17**:55. Available from: http://www.jbiomedsci.com/content/17/1/55. DOI: 10.1186/1423-0127-17-55

[55] Zamani M, Katebi M, Mehdizadeh M, et al. Coenzyme Q10 protects hippocampal neurons against ischemia/reperfusion injury via modulation of BAX/Bcl-2 expression. Basic and Clinical Neuroscience. 2012;**3**(5):5-10. Available from: http://bcn.iums.ac.ir/article-1-277-en.html

[56] Ditor DS, Bao F, Chen Y, et al. A therapeutic time window for anti-CD11d monoclonal antibody treatment yielding reduced secondary tissue damage and enhanced behavioral recovery following severe spinal cord injury. Journal of Neurosurgery. Spine. 2006;**5**(4):343-352. DOI: 10.3171/spi.2006.5.4.343

[57] Fleming JC, Bao F, Chen Y, et al. α4β1 integrin blockade after spinal cord injury decreases damage and improves neurological function. Experimental

Neurology. 2008;**214**:147-159. DOI: 10.1016/j.expneurol.2008.04.024

[58] Bao F, Chen Y, Schneider KA, et al. An integrin inhibiting molecule decreases oxidative damage and improves neurological function after spinal cord injury. Experimental Neurology. 2008;**214**:160-167. DOI: 10.1016/j.expneurol.2008.09.006

[59] Hauben E, Nevo U, Yoles E, et al. Autoimmune T cells as potential neuroprotective therapy for spinal cord injury. Lancet. 2000;**355**(9200):286-287. DOI: 10.1016/S0140-6736(99)05140-5

[60] Hauben E, Butovsky O, Nevo U, et al. Passive or active immunization with myelin basic protein promotes recovery from spinal cord contusion. The Journal of Neuroscience. 2000;**20**:6421-6430. DOI: 10.1523/JNEUROSCI.20-17-06421.2000

[61] Ibarra A, Hauben E. The therapeutic window after spinal cord injury can accommodate T cell-based vaccination and methylprednisolone in rats. The European Journal of Neuroscience. 2004;**19**(11):2984-2990. DOI: 10.1111/j.0953-816X.2004.03402.x

[62] Hauben E, Agranov E, Gothilf A, et al. Posttraumatic therapeutic vaccination with modified myelin self-antigen prevents complete paralysis while avoiding autoimmune disease. The Journal of Clinical Investigation. 2001;**108**:591-599. DOI: 10.1172/JCI12837

[63] Katsara M, Yuriev E, Ramsland PA, et al. Altered peptide ligands of myelin basic protein (MPB 87-99) conjugated to reduced mannan modulated immune response in mice. Immunology. 2009;**128**(4):521-533. DOI: 10.1111/j.1365-2567.2009.03137.x

[64] Barouch R, Schwartz M. Autoreactive T cells induce neurotrophin production by immune and neural cells in injured rat optic nerve: Implications for protective autoimmunity. The FASEB Journal. 2002;**16**(10):1304-1306. DOI: 10.1096/fj.01-0467fje

[65] Shaked I, Porat Z, Gersner R, et al. Early activation of microglia as antigen-presenting cells correlates with T cell-mediated protection and repair of the injured central nervous system. Journal of Neuroimmunology. 2004;**146**:84-93

[66] Wang Y, Li J, Kong P, et al. Enhanced expression of neurotrophic factors in the injured spinal cord through vaccination with myelin basic protein-derived peptide pulsed dendritic cells. Spine. 2015;**40**(2):95-101. DOI: 10.1097/BRS.0000000000000694

[67] Ibarra A, Sosa M, García E, et al. Prophylactic neuroprotection with A91 improves the outcome of spinal cord injured rats. Neuroscience Letters. 2013;**554**:59-63. DOI: 10.1016/j.neulet.2013.08.048

[68] Martiñón S, García E, Flores N, et al. Vaccination with a neural-derived peptide plus administration of glutathione improves the performance of paraplegic rats. The European Journal of Neuroscience. 2007;**26**(2):403-412. DOI: 10.1111/j.1460-9568.2007.05650.x

[69] Martiñón S, García E, Toscano D, et al. Long-term production of BDNF and NT-3 induced by A91-immunization after spinal cord injury. BMC Neuroscience. 2016;**17**(1):42. DOI: 10.1186/s12868-016-0267-6

[70] Suárez-Meade P, Malagón E, Herrera-Martínez E, et al. Uso de péptidos neurales modificados como tratamiento de una lesión en la médula espinal: Una visión general. Entreciencias. 2015;**3**(7):121-131 https://www.redalyc.org/articulo.oa?id=457644945001

[71] García E, Silva R, Flores R, et al. The severity of spinal cord injury determines the inflammatory gene expression pattern after immunization with neural-derived peptides. Journal of Molecular Neuroscience. 2018;**65**:190-195. DOI: 10.1007/s12031-018-1077-3

[72] Rodríguez R, Flores A, Fernández A, et al. Immunization with neural derived peptides plus scar removal induces a permissive microenvironment, and improves locomotor recovery after chronic spinal cord injury. BMC Neuroscience. 2017;**18**(1):7. DOI: 10.1186/s12868-016-0331-2

[73] Ibarra A, Mendieta E, Suarez P, et al. Motor recovery after chronic spinal cord transection: A proof-of-concept study evaluating a combined strategy. CNS & Neurological Disorders Drug Targets. 2018. DOI: 10.2174/187152731766618110 5101756

[74] Garrido O, Silva R, García E, et al. Therapeutic window for combination therapy of A91 peptide and glutathione allows delayed treatment after spinal cord injury. Basic & Clinical Pharmacology & Toxicology. 2013;**112**(5):314-318. DOI: 10.1111/ bcpt.12023

[75] Bermeo G, Ibarra A, García E, et al. Monocyte locomotion inhibitory factor produced by *E. histolytica* improves motor recovery and develops neuroprotection after traumatic injury to the spinal cord. BioMed Research International. 2013;**2013**:340727. DOI: 10.1155/2013/340727

[76] Giménez S, Pacheco M, Cruz E, et al. Ultrastructural changes associated with the inhibition of monocyte chemotaxis caused by products of axenically grown *Entamoeba histolytica*. Laboratory Investigation. 1987;**57**(1):45-51

[77] Rico G, Leandro E, Rojas S, et al. The monocyte locomotion inhibitory factor produced by *Entamoeba histolytica* inhibits induced nitric oxide production in human leukocytes. Parasitology Research. 2003;**90**(4):264-267. DOI: 10.1007/s00436-002-0780-7

[78] Kretschmer R, Rico G, Giménez S. A novel anti-inflammatory oligopeptide produced by *Entamoeba histolytica*. Molecular and Biochemical Parasitology. 2001;**112**(2):201-209. DOI: 10.1016/ S0166-6851(00)00367-4

[79] Morales M, Silva G, Soriano C, et al. The Cys-Asn-Ser carboxyl terminal end group is the pharmacophore of the amebic anti-inflammatory mnocyte locomotion inhibitory factor (MLIF). Molecular and Biochemical Parasitology. 2008;**158**(1):46-51. DOI: 10.1016/j. molbiopara.2007.11.010

[80] Barrientos C, Rico G, Giménez JA, et al. Computational study of the electronic structure characterization of a novel anti-inflammatory tripeptide derived from monocyte locomotion inhibitory factor (MLIF) pentapeptide. European Journal of Medicinal Chemistry. 2009;**44**(8):3114-3119. DOI: 10.1016/j.ejmech.2009.03.003

[81] Silva R, Estrada I, Ramos R, et al. The effect of anti-inflammatory pentapeptide produced by *Entamoeba histolytica* on gene expression in the U-937 monocytic line. Inflammation Research. 2008;**57**:145-150. DOI: 10.1007/s00011-007-6199-y

[82] Silva R, Morales M, Blanco F, et al. The monocyte locomotion inhibitory factor (MLIF) produced by *E. Histolytica* alters the expression of genes related to the wound-healing process. International Journal of Peptide Research and Therapeutics. 2012;**18**(4):391-401. DOI: 10.1007/ s10989-012-9315-7

[83] Velazquez J, Utrera D, Zentella A, et al. The amebic anti-inflammatory monocyte locomotion inhibitory factor

(MLIF) modifies the NF-kB nuclear translocation in human monocytes. European Cytokine Network. 2003;**14**:64-67

[84] Zhang Y, Chen J, Li F, et al. A pentapeptide monocyte locomotion inhibitory factor protects brain ischemia injury by targeting the eEF1A1/endothelial nitric oxide synthase pathway. Stroke. 2012;**43**(10):2764-2773. DOI: 10.1161/STROKEAHA.112.657908

[85] Giménez JA, Arenas E, Díaz L, et al. Effect of the monocyte locomotion inhibitory factor (MLIF) produced by *Entamoeba histolytica* on the expression of cell adhesion molecules (CAMs) in the skin of guinea pigs. Archives of Medical Research. 2000;**31**(4 suppl):92-93

[86] Xiaoping W, Chao W, Yan Y, et al. New monocyte locomotion inhibitory factor analogs protect against cerebral ischemia-reperfusión injury in rats. Bosnian Journal. 2017;**17**(23);221-227. DOI: 10.17305/bjbms.2017.1622

[87] Jiang S, Liu Y, Wang J. Cardioprotective effects of monocyte locomotion inhibitory factor on myocardial ischemic injury by targeting vimentin. Life Sciences. 2016;**15**(167): 85-91. DOI: 10.1016/j.lfs.2016.10.021

[88] Liu X, Hu P, Wang Y, et al. A validated UPLC-MS/MS method for the quantitation of an unstable peptide, monocyte locomotion inhibitory factor (MLIF) in human plasma and its application to a pharmacokinetic study. Journal of Pharmaceutical and Biomedical Analysis. 2018;**5**(157):75-83. DOI: 10.1016/j.jpba.2018.04.009

[89] Gaucher C, Boudier A, Bonetti J, et al. Glutathione: Antioxidant properties dedicated to nanotechnologies. Antioxidants. 2018;7:62. DOI: 10.3390/antiox7050062

[90] Grattagliano I, Vendemiale G, Lauterburg B. Reperfusion injury of the liver: Role of mitochondria and protection by glutathione ester. The Journal of Surgical Research. 1999;**86**:2-8. DOI: 10.1006/jsre.1999.5620

[91] Estrela J, Ortega A, Obrador E. Glutathione in cancer biology and therapy. Critical Reviews in Clinical Laboratory. 2006;**43**(2):143-181. DOI: 10.1080/10408360500523878

[92] Anderson M, Nilsson M, Eriksson P, et al. Glutathione monoethyl ester provides neuroprotection in a rat model stroke. Neuroscience Letters. 2004;**354**:163-165. DOI: 10.1016/j.neulet.2003.09.067

[93] Volodymyr I. Glutathione homeostasis and functions: potential targets for medical interventions. Journal of Amino Acids. 2012;**2012**, Article ID 736837, 26 p. DOI: 10.1155/2012/736837

[94] Odewumi C, Badisa V, Le U, et al. Protective effects of N-acetylcysteine against cadmium-induced damage in cultured rat normal liver cells. International Journal of Molecular Medicine. 2011;**27**(2):243-248. DOI: 10.3892/ijmm.2010.564

[95] Anderson M, Luo J. Glutathione therapy: From prodrugs to genes. Seminars in Liver Disease. 1998;**18**(4):415-424. DOI: 10.1055/s-2007-1007174

[96] Cacciatore I, Cornacchia C, Pinnen F, et al. Prodrug approach for increasing cellular glutathione levels. Molecules. 2010;**15**(3):1242-1264. DOI: 10.3390/molecules15031242

[97] Moses H, Brittany R, Andrea S, et al. Neuroproteomic study of nitrated proteins in moderate traumatic brain injury rats treated with gamma glutamyl cysteine ethyl ester administration post injury: Insight into the role of glutathione elevation in nitrosative stress. Proteomics: Clinical

Applications. 2016;**10**(12):1218-1224. DOI: 10.1002/prca.201600004

[98] Drake J, Kanski J, Varadarajan S, et al. Elevation of brain glutathione by γ-glutamylcysteine ethyl ester protects against peroxynitrite-induced oxidative stress. Journal of Neuroscience Research. 2002;**68**(6):776-784. DOI: 10.1002/jnr.10266

[99] Lok J, Leung W, Zhao S, et al. Gamma-glutamylcysteine ethyl ester protects cerebral endothelial cells during injury and decreases blood-brain barrier permeability after experimental brain trauma. Journal of Neurochemistry. 2011;**118**(2):248-255. DOI: 10.1111/j.1471-4159.2011.07294.x

[100] Guizar G, Ibarra A, Espitia A, et al. Glutathione monoethyl ester improves functional recovery, enhances neuron survival, and stabilizes spinal cord blood flow after spinal cord injury in rats. Neuroscience. 2005;**13**:639-649. DOI: 10.1016/j.neuroscience.2004.09.056

[101] Zhang Q, Yang H, An J, et al. Therapeutic effects of traditional Chinese medicine on spinal cord injury: A promising supplementary treatment in future. Hindawi Publishing Corporation Evidence-Based Complementary and Alternative Medicine. 2016;**2016**:18. Article ID 8958721. DOI: 10.1155/2016/8958721

[102] Sanli AM, Turkoglu E, Serbes G, et al. Effect of curcumin on lipid peroxidation, early ultrastructural findings and neurological recovery after experimental spinal cord contusion injury in rats. Turkish Neurosurgery. 2012;**22**(2):189-195. DOI: 10.5137/1019-5149.JTN.5193-11.1

[103] Margaill I, Plotkine M, Lerouet D. Antioxidant strategies in the treatment of stroke. Free Radical Biology and Medicine. 2005;**39**:429-443. DOI: 10.1016/j.freeradbiomed.2005.05.003

[104] Augusto O, Munzt V. EPR spin-trapping of protein radicals to investigate biological oxidative mechanisms. Amino Acids. 2007;**32**:535-542. DOI: 10.1007/s00726-006-0429-4

[105] Nash K, Rockenbauer A, Villamena F. Reactive nitrogen species reactivities with nitrones: Theoretical and experimental studies. Chemical Research in Toxicology. 2012;**25**:1581-1597. DOI: 10.1021/tx200526y

[106] Floyd R, Castro F, Zimmerman G, et al. Nitrone-based of neurodegenerative diseases. Their use alone or in combination with lanthionines. Free Radical Biology and Medicine. 2013;**62**:145-156. DOI: 10.1016/j.freeradbiomed.2013.01.033

[107] Gomez-Mejiba SE, Zhai Z, Della-Vedova MC et al. Immuno-spin trapping from biochemistry to medicine: Advances, challenges, and pitfalls. Focus in protein-centered radicals. Biochim Biophys Acta. 2013;**1840**(2):722-729. DOI: 10.1016/j.bbagen.2013.04.039

[108] Janzen EG, Poyer JL, et al. Biological spin trapping II. Toxicity of nitrone spin traps: Dose-ranging in the rat. Journal of Biochemical and Biophysical Methods. 1995;**30**:239-247. DOI: 10.1016/0165-022X(95)00012-1

[109] Shi H, Timmins G, Monske M, et al. Evaluation of spin trapping agents and trapping conditions for detection of cell-generated reactive oxygen species. Archives of Biochemistry and Biophysics. 2005;**437**:59-68. DOI: 10.1016/j.abb.2005.02.028

[110] Porcal W, Hernandez P, Ferreira A, et al. Heteroaryl nitrones as drugs for neurodegenerative diseases: Synthesis, neuroprotective properties, and free radicals scavenger properties. Journal of Medicinal Chemistry. 2008;**51**(19):6150-6159. DOI: 10.1021/jm8006432

[111] Chioua M, Sucunza D, Soriano E, et al. α-aryl-N-alkyl nitrones, as potential agents for stroke treatment: Synthesis, theoretical calculations, antioxidant, anti-inflammatory, neuroprotective, and brain-blood barrier permeability properties. Journal of Medicinal Chemistry. 2012;**55**:153-168. DOI: 10.1021/jm201105a

[112] López-González GV, Porcal-Quinta W. Estrés oxidativo/nitro-oxidativo como blanco terapéutico en enfermedades neurodegenerativas. OmniaScience. 2014:157-190. DOI: 10.3926/oms.43

[113] Oliveira C, Benfeito S, Fernandes C, et al. NO and HNO Donors, Nitrones, and Nitroxides: Past, Present, and Future. Wiley Online Library; Medicinal Research Reviews: 2017;**38**(4):1159-1187. DOI: 10.1002/med.21461

[114] Floy R, Kopke R, Choi C, et al. Nitrones as therapeutics. Free Radical Biology and Medicine. 2008;**45**(19):1361-1374. DOI: 10.1016/j.freeradbiomed.2008.08.017

[115] Hironobu Y, Nozomi I, Tohru Y, et al. Induction of neurite outgrowth by α-phenyl-N-tert-butylnitrone through nitric oxide release and Ras-ERK pathway in PC12 cells. Free Radical Research. 2010;**44**(6):645-654. DOI: 10.3109/10715761003692537

[116] Villamena F, Das N. Potential implication of chemical properties and bioactivity of nitrones spin traps for therapeutics. Future Medicinal Chemistry. 2012;**4**:1171-1207. DOI: 10.4155/fmc.12.74

[117] Tewari A, Mahendru V, Sinha A, et al. The new frontier for translational research in cerebroprotection. Journal of Anaesthesiology, Clinical Pharmacology. 2014;**30**(2):160-171. DOI: 10.4103/0970-9185.130001

[118] Chen G, Bray T, Janzen E, et al. Excretion, metabolism and tissue distribution of a spin trapping agent, alpha-phenyl-N-tert-butyl-nitrone (PBN) in rats. Free Radical Research Communications. 1990;**9**:317-323. DOI: 10.3109/10715769009145690

[119] Sang H, Wallis G, Stewart C, et al. Expression of cytokines and activation of transcription factors in lipopolysaccharide-administered rats and their inhibition by phenyl N tert-butylnitrone (PBN). Archives of Biochemistry and Biophysics. 1999;**363**:341-348. DOI: 10.1006/abbi.1998.1086

[120] Marklund N, Clausen F, Lewén A, et al. α-Phenyl-tert-N-butyl nitrone improves functional and morphological outcome after cortical contusion injury in the rat. Acta Neurochirurgica. 2001;**143**:73-81

[121] Sydserff S, Borelli A, Green A, et al. Effect of NXY-059 on infarct volume after transient or permanent middle cerebral artery occlusion in the rat; studies on dose, plasma concentration and therapeutic time window. British Journal of Pharmacology. 2002;**135**:103-112. DOI: 10.1038/sj.bjp.0704449

[122] Han M, He QP, Yong G, et al. NXY-059, a nitrone with free radical trapping properties inhibits release of cytochrome c after focal cerebral ischemia. Cellular and Molecular Biology. 2003;**49**:1249-1252

[123] Nash K, Ahmed S. Nanomedicine in the ROS-mediated pathophysiology: Applications and clinical advances. Nanomedicine. 2015;**11**:2033-2040. DOI: 10.1016/j.nano.2015.07.003

[124] Lees K, Barer D, Ford G, et al. Tolerability of NXY-059 at higher target concentrations in patients with acute stroke. Stroke. 2003;**34**:482-487. DOI: 10.1161/01.STR.0000053032.14223.81

[125] Zhai Z, Gómez S, Ramirez D. The nitrone spin

trap 5,5-dimethyl-1-pyrroline N-oxide affects stress response and fate of lipopolysaccharide-primed RAW264.7 macrophage cells. Inflammation. 2013;**36**:346-354. DOI: 10.1007/s10753-012-9552-4

[126] Hardy M, Chalier F, Ouari O, et al. Mito-DEPMPO synthesized from a novel NH_2-reactive DEPMPO spin trap: A new and improved trap for the detection of superoxide. Chemical Communications. 2007;**10**:1083-1085. DOI: 10.1039/B616076J

[127] Traynham C, Roof S, Wang H, et al. Diesterified nitrone rescues nitroso-redox levels and increases myocyte contraction via increased SR Ca(2+) handling. PLoS One. 2012;7(12):e52005. DOI: 10.1371/journal.pone.0052005

[128] Ban S, Nakagawa H, Suzuki T, et al. Novel mitochondria-localizing TEMPO derivative for measurement of cellular oxidative stress in mitochondria. Bioorganic & Medicinal Chemistry Letters. 2007;**17**:2055-2058. DOI: 10.1016/j.bmcl.2007.01.011

[129] Lee C, Yu L, Wang J. Nitroxide antioxidant as a potential strategy to attenuate the oxidative/nitrosative stress induced by hydrogen peroxide plus nitric oxide in cultured neurons. Nitric Oxide. 2016;**54**:38-50. DOI: 10.1016/j.niox.2016.02.001

[130] Deng Y, Singh I, Carrico K, et al. Neuroprotective effects of tempol, a catalytic scavenger of peroxynitrite-derived free radicals, in a mouse traumatic brain injury model. Journal of Cerebral Blood Flow and Metabolism. 2008;**28**:1114-1126. DOI: 10.1038/jcbfm.2008.10

[131] Hillard V, Peng H, Zhang Y, et al. Tempol, a nitroxide antioxidant, improves locomotor and histological outcomes after spinal cord contusion in rats. Journal of Neurotrauma. 2004;**21**:1405-1414. DOI: 10.1089/neu.2004.21.1405

[132] Francesco M, Paolo C, Oddose S, et al. Polyethylene glycol-superoxide dismutase, a conjugate in search of exploitation. Advanced Drug Delivery Reviews. 2002;**54**:587-606. DOI: 10.1016/S0169-409X(02)00029-7

[133] Shi R. Polyethylene glycol repairs membrane damage and enhances functional recovery: A tissue engineering approach to spinal cord injury. Neuroscience Bulletin. 2013;**29**(4):460-466. DOI: 10.1007/s12264-013-1364-5

[134] Kong X, Tang Q, Chen X, et al. Polyethylene glycol as a promising synthetic material for repair of spinal cord injury. Neural Regeneration Research. 2017;**12**(6):1003-1008. DOI: 10.4103/1673-5374.208597: 10.4103/1673-5374.208597

[135] Lu X, Perera T, Aria A, et al. Polyethylene glycol in spinal cord injury repairs: A critical review. Journal of Experimental Pharmacology. 2018;**10**:37-49. DOI: 10.2147/JEP.S148944

[136] Luo J, Borgens R, Shi R. Polyethylene glycol improves function and reduces oxidative stress in synaptosomal preparations following spinal cord injury. Journal of Neurotrauma. 2004;**21**(8):994-1007. DOI: 10.1089/0897715041651097

[137] Muizelaar J, Marmarou A, Young H, et al. Improving the outcome of severe head injury with the oxygen radical scavenger polyethylene glycol-conjugated superoxide dismutase: A phase II trial. Journal of Neurosurgery. 1993;**78**(3):375-382. DOI: 10.3171/jns.1993.78.3.0375

[138] He Y, Hsu C, Ezrin A, et al. Polyethylene glycol conjugated superoxide

dismutase in focal cerebral ischemia-reperfusion. American Journal of Physiology. 1993;**265**(1 Pt 2):H252-H256. DOI: 10.1152/ajpheart.1993.265.1.H252

[139] Wyn DN, Donald HK, Hasan BA, et al. Polyethylene glycol-superoxide dismutase inhibits lipid peroxidation in hepatic ischemia/reperfusion injury. Critical Care. 1999;**3**(5):127-130. DOI: 10.1186/cc358

[140] Granke K, Hollier L, Zdrahal P, et al. Longitudinal study of cerebral spinal fluid drainage in polyethylene glycol-conjugated superoxide dismutase in paraplegia associated with thoracic aortic cross-clamping. Journal of Vascular Surgery. 1991;**13**(5):615-621

[141] Edward D, Wang J, Miller D, et al. Newer pharmacological approach for antioxidant neuroprotection in traumatic brain injury. Neuropharmacology. 2018;**18**:30473-30478. DOI: 10.1016/j.neuropharm.2018.08.005

[142] Cruz J, Minoja G, Okuchi K. Improving clinical outcomes from acute subdural hematomas with the emergency preoperative administration of high doses of mannitol: A randomized trial. Neurosurgery. 2001;**49**:864-871

[143] Tenny S, Thorell W. Mannitol. Treasure Island (FL): StatPearls Publishing LLC; 2018. Bookshelf ID: NBK470392

[144] Grasner L, Winkler P, Strowitzki M, et al. Increased intrathecal pressure after traumatic spinal cord injury: An illustrative case presentation and a review of the literature. European Spine Journal. 2017;**26**(1):20-25. DOI: 10.1007/s00586-016-4769-9

[145] Reed J, Allen W, Dohrmann G. Effect of mannitol on the traumatized spinal cord. Microangiography, blood flow patterns, and electrophysiology. Spine. 1979;**4**(5):391-397

[146] De la Torre J, Johnson C, Goode D, et al. Pharmacologic treatment and evaluation of permanent experimental spinal cord trauma. Neurology. 1975;**25**(6):508-514

[147] Feldman Z, Reichenthal E, Zachari Z, et al. Mannitol, intracranial pressure, and Vasogenic Edema. Neurosurgery. 1995;**36**(6):1236-1237. DOI: 10.1227/00006123-199506000-00040

[148] Baysefer A, Erdogan E, Kahraman S, et al. Effect of mannitol in experimental spinal cord injury: An ultrastructural and electrophysiological study. Neurology India. 2003;**51**(3):350-354

[149] Parker A, Park R, Stowater J. Reduction of trauma-induced edema of spinal cord in dogs given mannitol. American Journal of Veterinary Research. 1973;**34**(10):1355-1357

[150] Salem N, Salem MY, Elmaghrabi MM, et al. Does vitamin C have the ability to augment the therapeutic effect of bone marrow-derived mesenchymal stem cells on spinal cord injury? Neural Regeneration Research. 2017;**12**(12):2050-2058. DOI: 10.4103/1673-5374.221163

[151] Aminmansour B, Asnaashari A, Rezvani M, et al. Effects of progesterone and vitamin D on outcome of patients with acute traumatic spinal cord injury: A randomized, double-blind, placebo controlled study. The Journal of Spinal Cord Medicine. 2016;**39**(3):272-280. DOI: 10.1080/10790268.2015.1114224

[152] Lee JY, Choi HY, Yune TY. Fluoxetine and vitamin C synergistically inhibits blood-spinal cord barrier disruption and improves functional recovery after spinal cord injury.

Neuropharmacology. 2016;**109**:78-87. DOI: 10.1016/j.neuropharm.2016.05.018

[153] Allison DJ, Thomas A, Beaudry K, et al. Targeting inflammation as a treatment modality for neuropathic pain in spinal cord injury: A randomized clinical trial. Journal of Neuroinflammation. 2016;**13**(1):152. DOI: 10.1186/s12974-016-0625-4

[154] Cordero K, Coronel GG, Serrano-Illán M, et al. Effects of dietary vitamin E supplementation in bladder function and spasticity during spinal cord injury. Brain Sciences. 2018;**8**(38):1-20. DOI: 10.3390/brainsci8030038

[155] Herrera García JS. Evaluation of motor recovery and gene expression from acute phase in rats with spinal cord injury [Master's thesis]. Mexico City, MX: National Autonomous University of Mexico; 2017

Chapter 5

Effects of Cyclosporin-A, Minocycline, and Tacrolimus (FK506) on Enhanced Behavioral and Biochemical Recovery from Spinal Cord Injury in Rats

Mohammad Ahmad and Abdualrahman Saeed Alshehri

Abstract

Spinal cord injury (SCI) results into an immediate primary injury (physical damages) followed by secondary damages (prolonged posttraumatic inflammatory disorder) resulting into severe motor dysfunction including paralysis. The present chapter discusses and investigates the neuroprotective effects of cyclosporin-A (CsA), minocycline, and tacrolimus (FK506) and their therapeutic effectiveness in recovery from the animal model of SCI. Based on the available recent literature on these three drugs, as well as in perspective of the results obtained on some experimental behavioral, biochemical, and oxidative stress parameters in the present study, the therapeutical potential of these three drugs has been discussed. Furthermore, the animal model of SCI used herein has been reviewed and compared with other reported animal models for understanding the utility, suitability, and reproducibility of the methodology of the present model for screening purposes in quest of searching ideal therapeutic compounds for maximum recovery from SCI.

Keywords: cyclosporin-A, minocycline, tacrolimus (FK506), rats, spinal cord injury, behavior, oxidative stress

1. Introduction

Spinal cord injury (SCI) is prevalent worldwide [1, 2] and often incapacitates the victims for life resulting in disability. Injury to the spinal cord results in processes that occur in three phases: the first phase is immediate physical phase also known as acute phase comprising affected spinal shock and initial trauma (primary injury) followed by the second phase known as secondary phase which is a prolonged cascade of damaging processes over a time period of minutes to weeks after the injury (secondary injury). Such damages include ischemia, vascular alterations, biochemical alterations, and cellular responses that lead to peripheral posttraumatic inflammatory cell infiltration and cell death (secondary injury) [1, 3–5]. The third phase that sustains between days and years after SCI trauma is characterized by proapoptotic degeneration and scarring that establishes permanent functional impairment [6, 7]. Secondary injury leads to the key pathophysiological response

 IntechOpen

to SCI causing severe and permanent functional deficits. Most of the clinical trials and experimental studies are conducted for intense research to unfold the underlying pathophysiological processes and for searching ideal and potential therapy for recovery from secondary SCI injuries [8]. Besides motor dysfunction, some of the other important SCI-related biochemical and immunological impairments that get involved are serum tumor necrosis factor (TNF)-α, interleukin (IL)-1β, interleukin-6, nuclear factor (NF)-κB p65, p38 mitogen-activated protein kinase (MAPK), inducible nitric oxide synthase (iNOS), caspase-3, superoxide dismutase (SOD), catalase (CAT), malondialdehyde (MDA), and glutathione peroxidase (GSH-Px) [9]. SCI trauma causes a devastating effect not only to the individual patient, but it also incurs heavy expensive burden to the society in general and to the family members, due to substantial long-term healthcare expenditures [10].

Despite considerable therapeutic studies, no proven drugs or techniques are available for satisfactory treatment of SCI. Much of these therapeutic studies have been reported from animal models, and it needs to be understood that a successful clinical trial in humans can only be initiated based on previously available preclinical data reported from animal model studies that closely mimic the losses as in human SCI functions [11]. Although rats are the animal model of choice for SCI studies, the major anatomical differences in axonal tracts and sensory motor pathways between quadrupeds and bipeds need to be taken into careful account to improve the targets of human SCI treatments [12].

Currently, methylprednisolone is the only recognized treatment for human SCI; however, it has significant adverse effects, including respiratory complications, sepsis, and gastrointestinal hemorrhage [13]. Furthermore, other important evidence-based therapies that have potential neuroprotective and neural reparative therapeutic properties and are undergoing clinical trials for human SCI include surgical decompression, blood pressure augmentation, riluzole, granulocyte colony-stimulating factor, minocycline, glibenclamide, cerebrospinal fluid drainage, magnesium, therapeutic hypothermia, Cethrin (VX-210), anti-NOGO antibody, cell-based approaches, and bioengineered biomaterials [5, 14, 15].

Some other experimental drugs that have been studied for therapeutical use in animal SCI are recombinant human erythropoietin [10], tetrodotoxin [16], BCL-2 [17], cyclosporin-A [18], edaravone [19], atorvastatin [20], calpain inhibitors [21] FK506, and minocycline [22]. Also, some natural products like eugenol oil [9], curcumin [23], and melatonin [24] have shown promising effects in animal SCI functional recovery. It sounds reasonable that instead of using a highly selective treatment that targets a specific molecule or pathway, a compound with multifunctional properties that targets several mediators involved in spinal cord pathology may be more effective for recovery from SCI [25]. In our earlier study [22], the promising potential of FK506 and minocycline has been reported for their effectiveness in rat SCI model. Thus, in the present study, besides these two multifactorial effective compounds minocycline and FK506, a third compound cyclosporin-A (CsA) was also included, and all the three compounds minocycline, FK506 (tacrolimus), and cyclosporine-A were chosen to evaluate in a comparative manner for their therapeutical potential using some important and reliable parameters that are most commonly used in rat SCI model [22]. Before discussing the outcome of our present results, we review the multifactorial effects of these three compounds that have been reported in literature using rat SCI model.

1.1 Minocycline

Minocycline, a semisynthetic second-generation tetracycline, has robust neuroprotective effects in rodent models of neurodegenerative diseases [26] and provides neuroprotection in experimental models of neurological diseases, including SCI [27]. In a broad range of secondary injury mechanisms via its anti-inflammatory, antioxidant, and antiapoptotic properties, minocycline is effective in reducing secondary injury and promoting locomotor functional recovery [28–31]. Minocycline prevents N-methyl-D-aspartate (NMDA)-induced excitotoxicity by diminishing NMDA-induced Ca^{2+} influx and mitochondrial Ca^{2+} uptake [32] and protects gray and white matter from SCI [33]. Minocycline also inhibits p38 mitogen-activated protein kinase (p38 MAPK) activation and microglial pro-nerve growth factor (proNGF) expression resulting from inflammatory reactions due to SCI and improves oligodendrocyte survival [34]. Inflammation due to SCI also upregulates and activates a class of enzymes like phospholipase A2s (PLA2s), and minocycline reduces cPLA2s [35]. It also inhibits monocyte and microglial expression of cyclooxygenase 2 (COX2) and production of proinflammatory prostaglandins E2 [36] and suppresses 5-lipoxygenase (5-LOX) action in SCI tissue [37]. Minocycline also eliminates free radicals in the post-SCI microenvironment and protects from oxidative stress [38]. It inhibits malondialdehyde, a by-product of lipid peroxidation [39, 40], and increases glutathione (GSH) [39], superoxide dismutase, and glutathione peroxidase [40], suggesting the powerful antioxidative mechanisms of minocycline to recover from secondary injury in SCI. Minocycline is reported to inhibit matrix metalloproteinases (MMPs) that are upregulated following SCI and are involved in injury and recovery processes [41, 42]. Furthermore, minocycline improves functional outcome, reduces lesion size and cell death, and alters cytokine expression after SCI [43–45]. Minocycline reduces the lesion area, increases the number of descending sympathoexcitatory axons traversing the injury site, and ultimately reduces the severity of autonomic dysreflexia [46]. In a murine model of SCI, minocycline treatment was superior to methylprednisolone in promoting functional improvement [44] and had neuroprotective effects on the SCI epicenter [47], motor neuron recovery, and neuropathic pain [48]. Minocycline has recently been reported to be effective in reducing secondary injury and promoting locomotor functional recovery in experimental SCI [28].

It has also been reported to attenuate reactive astrocytosis in SCI which directly damages cell bodies and triggers endogenous processes including neuroinflammation and reactive astrocytosis [49, 50]. In combination studies also, minocycline has been reported for better recovery from SCI when used in combination with other drugs like FK506 [22] and bone marrow mesenchymal cells (BMSCs) [51] showing a very significant recovery in behavioral function, oxidative stress, and reduction in lesion size from SCI in rats warranting further research on this drug.

1.2 Cyclosporin-A

Cyclosporin-A is an immunosuppressive cyclic undecapeptide that inhibits T cells and depresses both cellular and humoral immune responses to prevent graft rejection and reduces the inflammatory responses [52]. CsA significantly decreases the expression levels of interleukin-10, tumor necrosis factor-α, cyclophilin-D (Cyp-D), and apoptosis-inducing factor (AIF) [53]. CsA does not readily cross the blood-spinal cord barrier (BSCB), which restricts the clinical application of CsA for SCI treatment. Thus, polyethylene glycol (PEG)-transactivating-transduction protein (TAT)-modified CsA-loaded cationic multifunctional polymeric liposome-poly (lactic-co-glycolic acid) (PLGA) core/shell nanoparticles (PLGA/CsA NPs) to transport and deliver CsA across the BSCB have a new potential to treat SCI [54]. CsA inhibits primarily the inflammatory reaction and the synthesis of constitutive nitric oxide (NO) and inducible nitric oxide synthases (NOS), well-known neurotoxic agents for SCI diminishing overproduction of free radicals, and secondarily lipid peroxidation (LP) observed after SCI [55, 56]. CsA may also induce other non-immunological effects that could be beneficial for treatment of neurological disorders [57]. CsA has been widely used in the treatment of various diseases including aplastic anemia, nephritic syndrome, rheumatoid arthritis, psoriasis, and cerebral ischemic injuries [53]. CsA promotes neuroprotection by diminishing both demyelination and neuronal cell death, resulting in a better motor outcome after SCI [52, 58, 59]. CsA in combination with FK506 had a neuroprotective treatment against SCI hypoxia-induced damage mediated via their antioxidant actions on mitochondrial ATP, tissue-reduced glutathione, tissue LPO level, and myeloperoxidase (MPO) activity [60]. Administration of CsA in combination with olfactory ensheathing cell (OEC) transplantation results in augmented functional improvements and promotes axon regeneration after SCI [61].

1.3 FK506

FK506 (tacrolimus), a macrolide lactane antibiotic, was introduced as an immunosuppressive agent [62] with virtually no side effects [63]. FK506, a potent calcineurin inhibitor, exhibits neuroprotective actions in several experimental models of central nervous system trauma, including stroke, and improved neurological recovery following peripheral and spinal cord injuries [47, 63–67]. It is reported that FK506 has beneficial effects in SCI recovery involving various mechanisms such as neuroregeneration and neuroprotection [67], promotion of axonal outgrowth [68], and suppression of oxidative stress [60]. FK506 improves the functional outcome of SCI [67–69] and has an in vivo neurotrophic action, whereby it enhances the rate of axon regeneration, leading to more rapid neurological recovery [70–73]. Significant functional recovery from SCI due to FK506 treatment has been reported in rat models [22, 67, 74]. Activation of NF-κB and proinflammatory cytokines (TNF-a, IL-1b, and IL-6) expression levels in SCI animals is reversed by FK506 treatment involving microglial activation after SCI [7]. FK506 upregulates epidermal growth factor (EGF)-level expression of astrocytes that have an important role as mediators for SCI functional recovery promoting axonal regeneration [74]. FK506 in combination as a cocktail with other drugs like minocycline [22], CSA [60], RhoA inhibitors [75], nerve growth factor (NFG) [76], and methylprednisolone (MP) [77] has shown significant therapeutic recovery from SCI in rats.

Considering the above-discussed multifactorial effects of CsA, minocycline, and FK506, the present study was undertaken to investigate the neuroprotective effects of these three compounds in a comparative manner on recovery from experimental SCI, as these three drugs target multiple processes involved in mediating cell death and the development of secondary injury in SCI. Furthermore, our earlier findings on FK506 and minocycline [22] prompted us to include CsA (another promising drug for SCI recovery) and compare their effectiveness in rat model of SCI, using the behavioral and biochemical parameters as in earlier [22].

2. Utility of experimental animal models for SCI studies

For SCI studies, animal models are used because of their easy accessibility, convenience, and capability of the researchers to explore them at several levels (simulated to human clinical SCI levels) for motor functional, biochemical, and oxidative stress and genetic, therapeutic, and pathophysiological evaluations [78]. Over the last decade, a variety of animal models have been used for experimental SCI studies, including rats, mice, gerbils, guinea pigs, hamsters, rabbits, dogs, goats, pigs, and nonhuman primates [79]. Among these animals, rodents in general and rats in particular are the most widely and commonly studied SCI models [80]. In the present study also, we have used young adult male Sprague-Dawley rats with all similar specifications of breeding, housing facilities, and experimental handlings, as described in our earlier study [22].

To establish an ideal SCI animal model for research purposes, various models have been tried and reported till to date in quest of searching methodology to obtain maximum recovery from SCI. These experimental animal models include spinal cord traumatic injury model [81], photochemical-induced SCI model [82], spinal cord transection model [83], bidirectional distraction SCI model [84], and the spinal cord ischemia-reperfusion injury model [85]. For traumatic injury model, the contusive SCI model is used by inducing contusion on the dorsal spinal cord by dropping a desired weight either from a computer-controlled impact device [86] or from a customized impact device [87]. Another traumatic injury model known as compressive SCI model is also very commonly used where instead of dropping the weight, it is placed on the exposed spinal cord segment in the dorsoventral direction to induce a compressive SCI [88, 89]. However, since SCI caused by impact and compression is more common in clinical patients [79], in the present study also, we have used the compressed SCI model induced in the rats as described in our earlier study [22]. Briefly, the SCI was induced in the rats following the modified method of Nystrom and Berglund [89]. Laminectomy was performed at the T 7–8 level, and spinal cord compression injury was produced by placing a load with a total weight of 35 g, for 5 min over the exposed extradural area.

All experimental rats were randomly divided into the following six groups with eight animals in each as described earlier [22]:

Group I: The normal control group without laminectomy or compression injury

Group II: Sham group with laminectomy alone but no spinal compression injury

Group III: SCI control group with laminectomy and spinal compression injury

SCI-treated groups were the same as the SCI control group (Group III) and consisted of three groups in which the effect on the recovery from SCI using the same parameters is mentioned in our earlier study [22]. Doses of the three drugs CSA, minocycline, and FK506 were selected on the basis of our pilot screening of these drugs at low, medium, and high doses, and the best effective dose in each was used in the present study as follows:

Group IV: Cyclosporin-A 5 mg/kg

Group V: Minocycline 50 mg/kg

Group VI: FK506 (tacrolimus) 1 mg/kg

All protocols for the drug administration, follow-ups, care, and experimental handlings of the animals for various evaluation parameters were the same as described earlier [22].

3. Behavioral evaluations in SCI animals

To analyze the therapeutic recovery from induced SCI in animal models, several behavioral outcome measures have been developed and widely used, such as the catwalk [90], the Basso-Beattie-Bresnahan (BBB) locomotor scale [91], the horizontal ladder test, and the cylinder rearing test [92]. From the literature review of the recent years, it is found that BBB locomotor scale has been most widely used in SCI rat models to evaluate motor functional recovery from SCI [9, 12, 22–24, 53, 58, 74, 77, 93]. However, in the present study, besides BBB locomotor scale [94], a battery of some more behavioral motor functions was included like Tarlov scoring [95], inclined plane test [96], and some functional deficit scorings like toe spread, platform hang, wire mesh descent, and hind foot bar grab [97, 98]. Our pilot study showed that a naive control group of animals treated with CsA, minocycline, and FK506 without SCI showed no different behaviors than the naïve control untreated groups (data not shown in behavioral results) for all the observed behavioral parameters. Thus, the results of the drug treatments alone were not included in all behavioral results (**Figures 1–4**).

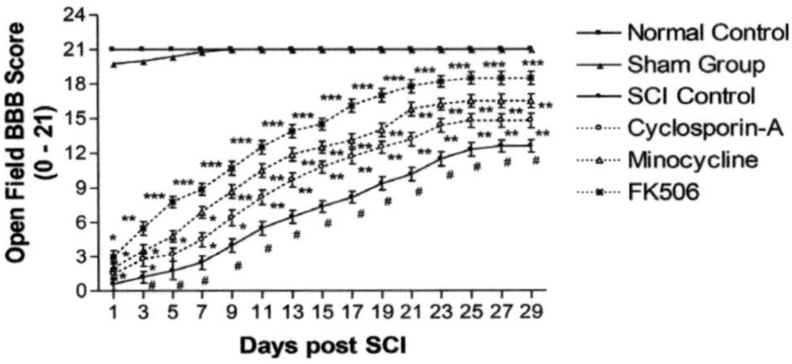

Figure 1.
*Effect of CSA, FK506, and minocycline on gait performance tunnel (GPT) behavioral motor performance activities (BBB Score) of hind limbs of rats subjected to SCI. The graph shows the comparative functional recovery from SCI over a period of 29 days. Animals were treated with the drugs daily after SCI for 3 weeks. Abbreviations: CSA, cyclosporin-A; FK506, tacrolimus; SCI, spinal cord injury; BBB, Basso, Beattie, and Bresnahan. Drug doses used are cyclosporin (5 mg/kg), FK506 (1 mg/kg), and minocycline (50 mg/kg); the drugs are effective in the order FK506 > minocycline > cyclosporin-A. # shows the SCI group is significantly ($p < 0.001$) different from the SCI uninjured control group. *, **, and *** represent the SCI-treated groups are significantly different at $p < 0.05$, $p < 0.01$, and $p < 0.001$, respectively, compared to the SCI group by ANOVA with post hoc testing using Tukey-Kramer or Student-Newman-Keuls Multiple Comparison Tests.*

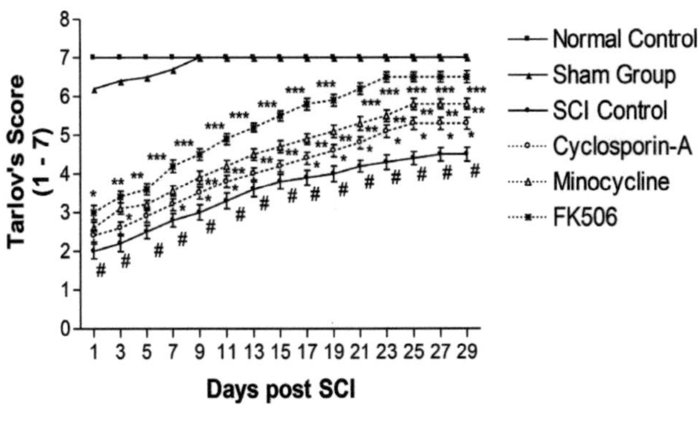

Figure 2.
The effect of cyclosporin-A, FK506, and minocycline on the behavioral motor performance activity (Tarlov's Score) of hind limbs of rats subjected to SCI. The graph shows the comparative functional recovery from SCI over a period of 29 days. Animals were treated with drugs daily after SCI for 3 weeks. Abbreviations, drugs used and their doses, and all statistical significances are the same as in **Figure 1**.

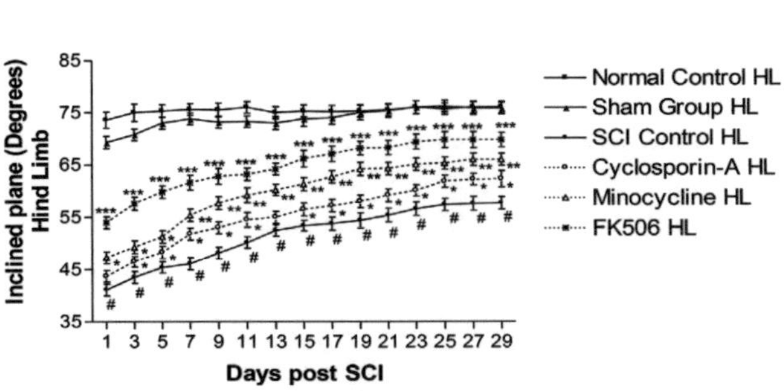

Figure 3.
The effect of cyclosporin-A, FK506, and minocycline on the behavioral motor performance activity (Inclined Plane Test) of hind limbs (HL) of rats subjected to SCI. The graph shows the comparative functional recovery from SCI over a period of 29 days. Animals were treated with drugs daily after SCI for 3 weeks. Abbreviations, drugs used and their doses, and all statistical significances are the same as in **Figure 1**.

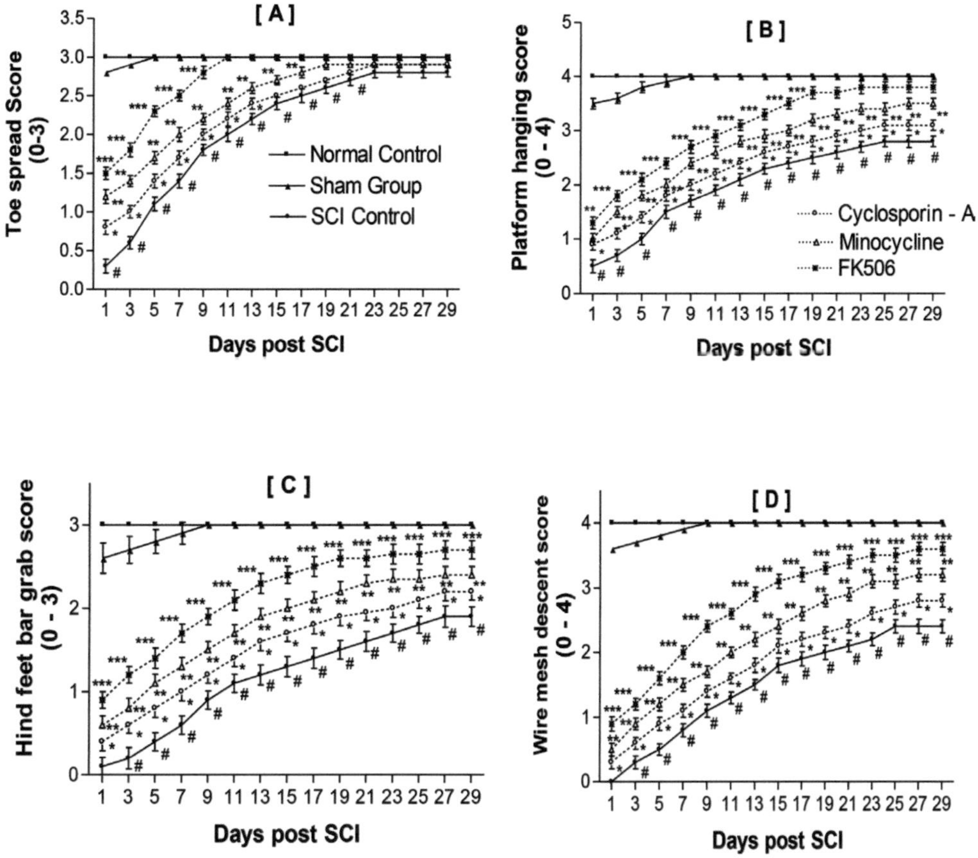

Figure 4.
(A–D) The effect of cyclosporin-A, FK506, and minocycline on the behavioral motor functional scoring of toe spread (A), platform hanging (B), hind foot bar grab (C), and wire mesh decent (D) of rats subjected to SCI. The graph shows the comparative functional recovery from SCI over a period of 29 days. Animals were treated with drugs daily after SCI for 3 weeks. Abbreviations, drugs used and their doses, and all statistical significances are the same as in **Figure 1**.

The present results of behavioral observations indicated that treatment with all the three drugs in this study induced significant recovery from SCI with respect to time in all behavioral activities compared to the SCI control group, and the drugs were effective in the order of FK506 > minocycline > CsA ($F = 13.49$, $F = 5.82$, and $F = 3.14$; $df = 3$; $p < 0.001$, $p < 0.01$, and $p < 0.05$, respectively) throughout (**Figures 1–4**).

4. Biochemical evaluations in SCI animal models

Biochemical evaluations have a vast list of parameters that exist as biomarkers for assessing recovery from SCI in animal models. Some of the most important biochemical parameters include oxidative stress indices like lipid peroxidation and total glutathione, nitric oxide synthase, myeloperoxidase, mitochondrial permeability, inflammatory responses, autonomic dysreflexia, cerebrospinal fluid biomarkers, immune responses, astrocyte modulations, etc., and all of these have been reviewed in detail earlier in this chapter, especially for the three drugs, CsA, minocycline, and FK506, that have been evaluated in the present study.

The biochemical parameters evaluated in this study included determination of monoamines 5-hydroxy-indoleacetic acid (5-HIAA) and serotonin or 5-hydroxy tryptamine (5-HT) [99], lipid peroxides determined as thiobarbituric acid-reactive substances (TBARS) [100, 101], total glutathione [102, 103], and myeloperoxidase [104] and have been described for their methods in our earlier study [22].

The present biochemical results showed significant ameliorating effect of all three drugs on the levels of 5-HT (**Figure 5A**, 5-HIAA; **Figure 5B**, on the ratio of 5-HIAA; and **Figure 5C**, 5-HT). TBARS was significantly stimulated (**Figure 6A**), whereas GSH was significantly inhibited (**Figure 6B**), and MPO level was significantly diminished toward the normal level (**Figure 6C**). Overall, the entire biochemical parameters evaluated in the present study were significantly affected by the three drugs effectively in the order FK506 > minocycline > CsA throughout.

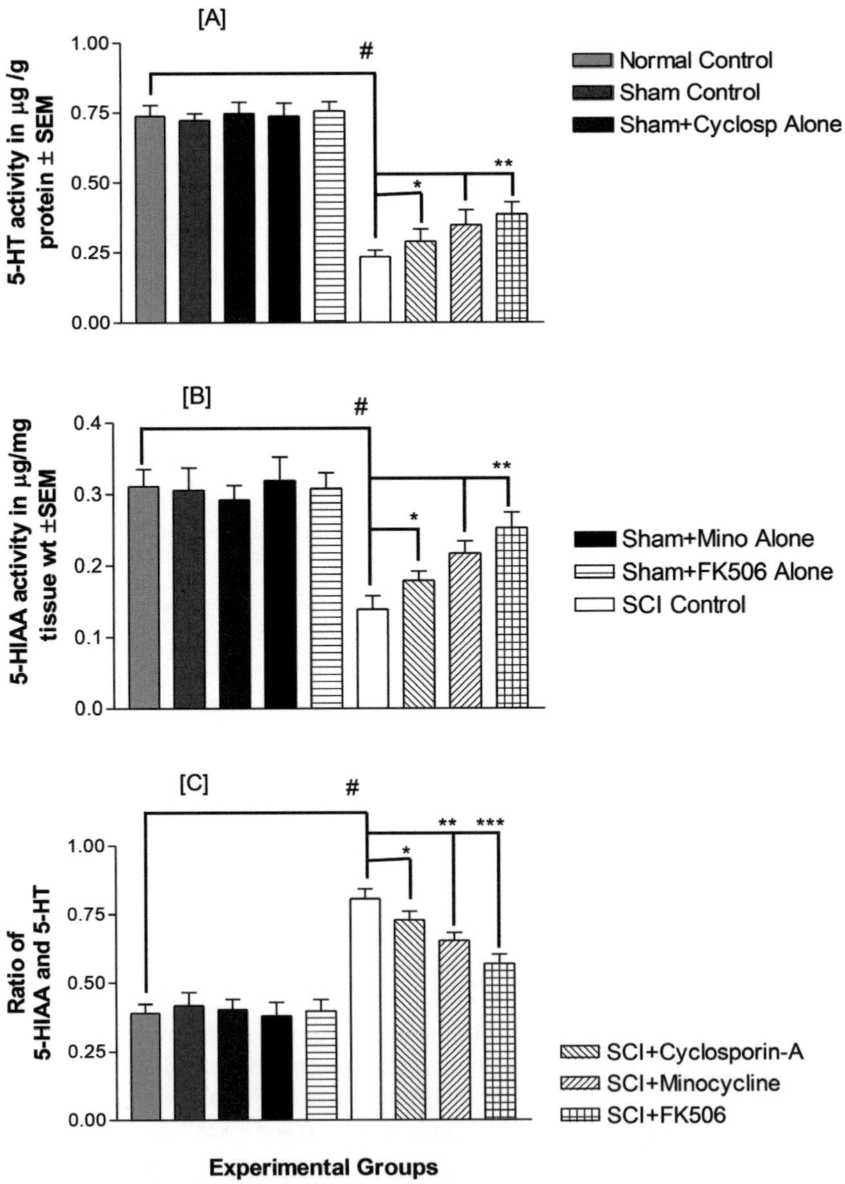

Figure 5.
(A–C) Levels of (A) 5-HT (5-hydroxytryptamine), (B) 5-HIAA (5-hydroxy-indoleacetic acid), and (C) the ratio of 5-HIAA and 5-HT activities in the spinal cord tissue of rats 29 days post-SCI and the effects of treatment with various drugs. Abbreviations, drugs used and their doses, and all statistical significances are the same as in **Figure 1.**

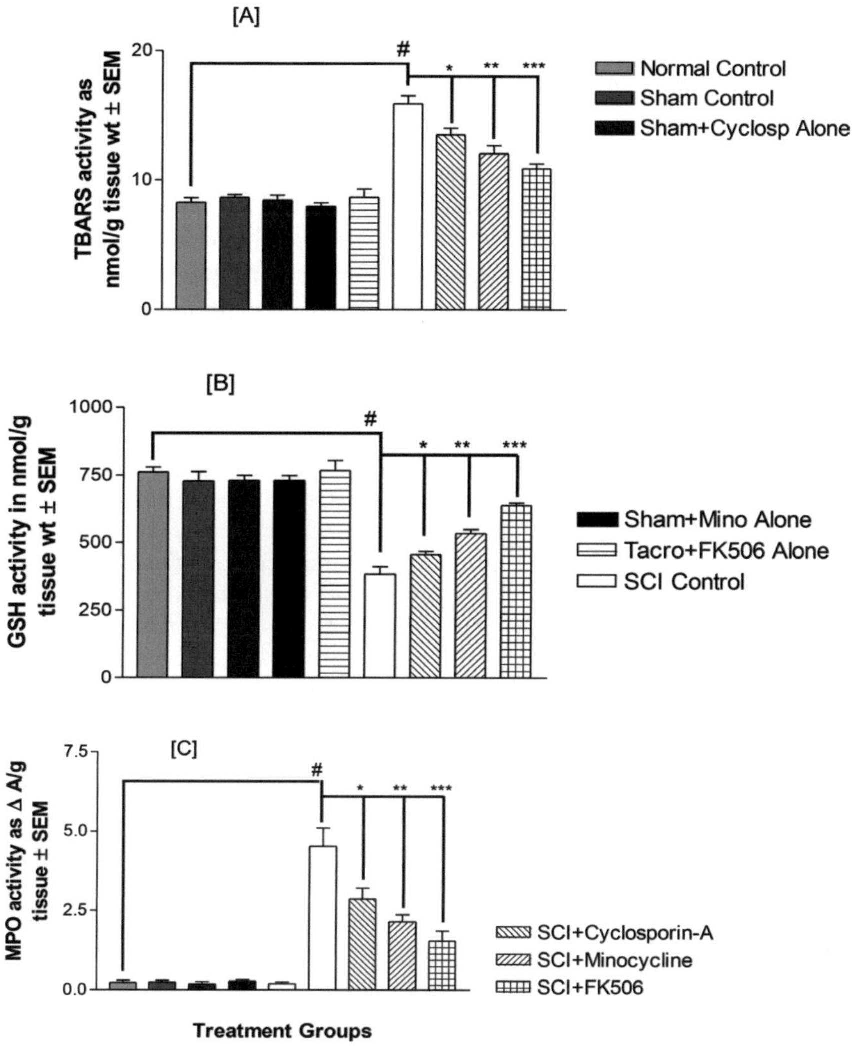

Figure 6.
Levels of (A) thiobarbituric acid, (B) glutathione, and (C) myeloperoxidase activities in the injured spinal cord tissue of rats 29 days post-SCI and the effects of treatment with various drugs. Abbreviations, drugs used and their doses, and all statistical significances are the same as in **Figure 1**.

5. Discussion

SCI leads to persistent pain and motor dysfunction, both of which lack effective therapeutics [105]. Therapeutic approaches that promote both neuroprotection and neuroregeneration are valuable for SCI therapies [52]. From the present discussed literature, the potential agents that have generated interest in SCI studies in the recent past include the multifactorial drugs minocycline, FK506, and CsA [18, 22, 52, 106].

In the present chapter also, the treated rats showed recovery in their hind limb reflexes rapidly regaining responses comparable with those of uninjured control rats (**Figure 1**). Although all drug-treated groups showed improved recovery in BBB and all behavioral activities, the best and the most significant recovery was observed with FK506 treatment. The drugs were effective in the order FK506 > minocycline > CsA throughout. Earlier studies have also used BBB scoring along with other behavioral parameters and have shown significant behavioral functional outcome in the

SCI animals treated with FK506 [7, 22, 60, 67, 69, 70, 74, 76], minocycline [22, 28, 43–45], and CsA [18, 52, 53, 58, 61]. In addition to the therapeutic effects of the three drugs, it has been also suggested that the daily routine behavioral assessment procedures may also assist the animals as equivalent to their exercises that help them to recover from SCI [107]. However, more studies are required to confirm this presumption. Additionally, no notable side effects were noted at the dosing regimen of the drugs (selected from the pilot studies) used in the present chapter. However, it has been suggested particularly for FK506 [63] that the therapeutic dosing regimen is a key factor that can affect efficacy as a neuroprotectant for CNS injuries.

FK506 has been reported by others also for being a potential therapy for SCI recovery through various mechanisms [7, 60, 63, 68, 108]. It is evidently proven that FK506 prevents the activation of NF-κB in microglia which reduces production of proinflammatory cytokines like TNF-a, IL-1b, and IL-6 in the SCI responses for effective recovery [7, 109]. Furthermore, it is suggested that inhibition of inflammatory reaction in SCI by FK506 could be due to its inhibitory action on decreasing the free radical formation and lipid peroxidation preventing calcineurin-mediated dephosphorylation of NOS activity in a Ca^{2+}-dependent manner [77]. FK506 also enhances neurite outgrowth and improves functional recovery from SCI by stimulating astrocytes to secrete epidermal growth factor (EGF) for neural repair [74].

CsA has also been reviewed and reported as a potent neuroprotectant for functional recovery from SCI [5, 55]. The significant protective role of CsA has been reported for recovery from SCI through inhibiting the apoptosis of spinal cord cells [53], improving locomotor function [58], increasing mean arterial pressure [110], inhibiting NOS [56], diminishing demyelination and neuronal cell death [60], attenuating reactive astrocytosis due to injury improved neurologic outcome [50], and reducing pain [111].

Minocycline has also been reviewed recently for its effectiveness through multiple mechanisms for functional recovery from SCI [38]. The multiple targets that minocycline works for SCI functional recovery include upregulation of the protein VEGF and BDNF expressions; downregulation of protein p-38MAPK, proNGF, p75NTR, and RhoA expressions and suppressed caspase-3 activity [51]; and improved antioxidant activity through amelioration in oxidative stress in the SCI tissue [40].

Monoamines such as norepinephrine (NE), dopamine (DA), and serotonin (5-HT) can activate the spinal neurons involved in walking [112–114]. Thus, the decrease in the level of 5-HT and 5-HIAA in the SCI animals in the present chapter clearly indicates that SCI inevitably affects the normal functioning of these spinal neurotransmitters involved in locomotor function. SCI-injured animals treated with the drugs herein improved levels of 5-HT and 5-HIAA (**Figure 5A–C**, respectively). Our present behavioral findings also showed an overall correlation and significant improvement in the functional deficits of the hind limbs after treatment with these drugs, indicating the presence of potential mechanisms of serotonergic agents in these drugs, as present in indorenate (5-methoxytryptamine, beta-methyl carboxylate hydrochloride), a 5-HT1A agonist that improved motor function in rats with chronic SCI [115].

The oxidant/antioxidant balance was clearly reflected by the increased level of TBARS (**Figure 6A**) and decreased level of GSH (**Figure 6B**) in the contused tissue of SCI control animals. However, treatment of SCI animals with the drugs interfered with the formation of free radicals following traumatic SCI. The comparative behavioral restorative effects of these drugs in the formation of free radicals in injured SC were in the order of FK506 > minocycline > CsA.

Spinal cord injury in mice results in severe trauma characterized by edema and neutrophil infiltration (measured as an increase in myeloperoxidase activity), and these neutrophils are thought to be involved in tissue injury through the release of various inflammatory mediators [116, 117]. The MPO levels in the present SCI animals were also significantly increased in the injured spinal cord tissue (**Figure 6C**). However, administration of minocycline, FK506, and CsA interfered significantly with the formation of MPO following traumatic SCI. The comparative restorative effects of these drugs in the formation of MPO in injured SC were in the order of FK506 > minocycline > CsA.

The pathophysiological events resulting from SCI are reported to involve free radical production; lipid peroxidation; excitotoxic molecules such as glutamate, eicosanoid, and prostaglandin production; protease activity; and intracellular increases in Ca^{2+} [118]. Furthermore, the primary auto-destructive event is initiated by the hydrolysis of fatty acids from membrane phospholipids, leading to cellular damage [119], and microglia becomes activated [120], which in turn may release neurotoxic molecules that further damage nearby neurons [121].

The hind limb functional deficits in the model of SCI (like the one as in the present chapter) are largely due to the loss of white matter axonal tracts [16, 122]. The white matter degeneration is caused by the primary injury (i.e., mechanical lesion), and there is also evidence that post-SCI demyelination caused by oligodendrocyte death/malfunction contributes significantly to chronic SCI functional deficits [123, 124].

The secondary injury is reported to result from several proposed auto-destructive events, including reactive oxygen species-induced lipid peroxidation [125], activation of non-NMDA ionotropic glutamate receptors [126], and caspase-3 activation [127, 128]. Secondary injury events include Na^{+} influx-mediated intra-axonal Ca^{+} accumulation leading to proteinase activation, which destroys the cytoskeleton [16, 129], as well as the induction of oligodendroglial apoptosis with subsequent demyelination of the surviving axons [79, 130]. Lipid peroxidation is one of the main pathological mechanisms involved in secondary damage after SCI [79]. Another key factor in the secondary injury mechanism is Ca^{2+} ions. Following trauma or ischemia, Ca^{2+} influx plays an important role in the pathogenesis of neural injury [130, 131]. Many drugs, including steroids, gangliosides, ion channel blockers, antioxidants, and free radical scavengers, have mild therapeutic effectiveness in experimental spinal cord injury [74, 119]. Another mechanism to promote functional recovery after spinal cord injury is enhancing axonal regeneration. Several strategies, including blocking myelin or glial scar inhibitors, delivery of neurotrophic factors, and cell transplantation, induce axonal outgrowth after experimental spinal cord injury. Among them, olfactory ensheathing cell grafts promote neuroprotection, axonal regeneration, and functional recovery after incomplete spinal cord injury [132, 133]. Furthermore, a regular enforced movement activity may additionally help provide faster functional restoration and recovery after SCI [134].

Studies on combinatorial effects of CsA, minocycline, and FK506 in various combinations with each other or with other compounds may prove to be more effective in recovery from SCI. Earlier combined treatments like FK506 and NGF [76], FK506 and minocycline [22], FK506 and methylprednisolone [77], FK506 and RhoA inhibitor [76, 77], minocycline and bone marrow mesenchymal stem cells [51], and CsA with PEG-TAT [54] have all shown significant functional recovery from SCI as compared to these compounds individually.

6. Conclusions

From the overall literature review on the multifactorial effects of CsA, minocycline, and FK506 and from the discussion of the present findings, it can be concluded that the drugs CsA, minocycline, and FK506 induce good recovery from experimentally induced SCI in rats. However, these drugs significantly improve functional restoration, replenish 5-HT and 5-HIAA levels, and restore the oxidant/antioxidant balance in the contused tissue after moderate SCI in rats in the order FK506 < minocycline < CsA. Furthermore, it is suggested that the present compressive SCI model of rats could still serve as the most convenient model for therapeutic screenings of various drugs in search of ideal therapy for SCI. CsA, minocycline, and FK506 appear to have gained support in a multifactorial effective manner through ample research work and should be considered as ideal therapeutical agents for the treatment of acute SCI. These drugs should be supported for clinical trials with further studies and tests. Although FK506 appears to be the most promising among the three drugs, more work is needed to screen all three compounds as cocktails in various combinations with better expected outcomes in SCI recovery possibly due to their cumulative multifactorial beneficial effects.

Acknowledgements

The authors are thankful to the Deanship of Scientific Research, College of Nursing Research Centre at King Saud University, for funding this research.

Conflict of interest

The authors have no conflict of interests.

Author details

Mohammad Ahmad* and Abdualrahman Saeed Alshehri
Department of Medical Surgical Nursing, College of Nursing,
King Saud University, Riyadh, Saudi Arabia

*Address all correspondence to: mbadshah@ksu.edu.sa

References

[1] Sekhon LH, Fehlings MG. Epidemiology, demographics, and pathophysiology of acute spinal injury. Spine (Phila Pa 1976). 2001;**26**:S2-S12

[2] Saunders LL, Clarke A, Tate DG, Forchheimer M, Krause JS. Lifetime prevalence of chronic health conditions among persons with spinal cord injury. Archives of Physical Medicine and Rehabilitation. 2015;**96**:673-679. DOI: 10.1016/j.apmr.2014.11.019

[3] O'Brien MF, Lenke LG, Lou J, Bridwell KH, Joyce ME. Astrocyte response and transforming growth factor-beta localization in acute spinal cord injury. Spine (Phila Pa 1976). 1994;**19**:2321-2329

[4] Gorman PH. The review of systems in spinal cord injury and dysfunction. Continuum (Minneapolis, Minn.). 2001;**17**:630-634. DOI: 10.1212/01.CON.0000399092.88866.1c

[5] Ahuja CS, Nori S, Tetreault L, Wilson J, Kwon B, Harrop J, et al. Traumatic spinal cord injury-repair and regeneration. Neurosurgery. 2017;**80**: 9-22. DOI: 10.1093/neuros/nyw080

[6] Profyris C, Cheema SS, Zang D, Azari MF, Boyle K, Petratos S. Degenerative and regenerative mechanisms governing spinal cord injury. Neurobiology of Disease. 2004;**15**:415-436. DOI: 10.1016/j.nbd.2003.11.015

[7] Liu G, Fan G, Guo G, Kang W, Wang D, Xu B, et al. FK506 attenuates the inflammation in rat spinal cord injury by inhibiting the activation of NF-κB in microglia cells. Cellular and Molecular Neurobiology. 2017;**37**:843-855. DOI: 10.1007/s10571-016-0422-8

[8] Thuret S, Moon LD, Gage FH. Therapeutic interventions after spinal cord injury. Nature Reviews. Neuroscience. 2006;**7**:628-643. DOI: 10.1038/nrn1955

[9] Ma L, Mu Y, Zhang Z, Sun Q. Eugenol promotes functional recovery and alleviates inflammation, oxidative stress, and neural apoptosis in a rat model of spinal cord injury. Restorative Neurology and Neuroscience. 2018;**36**:659-668. DOI: 10.3233/RNN-180826

[10] Gorio A, Gokmen N, Erbayraktar S, Yilmaz O, Madaschi L, Cichetti C, et al. Recombinant human erythropoietin counteracts secondary injury and markedly enhances neurological recovery from experimental spinal cord trauma. Proceedings of the National Academy of Sciences of the United States of America. 2002;**99**:9450-9455. DOI: 10.1073/pnas.142287899

[11] Lukovic D, Moreno-Manzano V, Lopez-Moncholi E, Rodriguez-Jime'nez FJ, Jendelova P, Sykova E, et al. Complete rat spinal cord transection as a faithful model of spinal cord injury for translational cell transplantation. Scientific Reports. 2015;**5**:9640. DOI: 10.1038/srep09640

[12] Filipp ME, Travis BJ, Henry SS, Idzikowski EC, Magnuson SA, Loh MY, et al. Differences in neuroplasticity after spinal cord injury in varying animal models and humans. Neural Regeneration Research. 2019;**14**:7-19. DOI: 10.4103/1673-5374.243694

[13] Fu ES, Tummala RP. Neuroprotection in brain and spinal cord trauma. Current Opinion in Anaesthesiology. 2005;**18**:181-187. DOI: 10.1097/01.aco.0000162838.56344.88

[14] Witiw CD, Fehlings MG. Acute Spinal Cord Injury. Journal of Spinal Disorders & Techniques. 2015;**28**:202-210. DOI: 10.1097/BSD.0000000000000287

[15] Uindreaj A, Badner A, Fehlings MG. Promising neuroprotective strategies for traumatic spinal cord injury with a focus on the differential effects among anatomical levels of injury. F1000Res. 2017;**6**:1907. DOI: 10.12688/f1000research.11633.1

[16] Teng YD, Wrathall JR. Local blockade of sodium channels by tetrodotoxin ameliorates tissue loss and long-term functional deficits resulting from experimental spinal cord injury. The Journal of Neuroscience. 1997;**17**:4359-4366

[17] Seki T, Hida K, Tada M, Koyanagi I, Iwasaki Y. Role of the bcl-2 gene after contusivespinal cord injury in mice. Neurosurgery. 2003;**53**:192-198

[18] Ibarra A, Correa D, Willms K, Merchant MT, Guizar-Sahagun G, Grijalva I. Effects of cycolsporin-A on immune response, tissue protection and motor function of rats subjected to spinal cord injury. Brain Research. 2003;**979**:165-178

[19] Ohta S, Iwashita Y, Takada H, Kuno S, Nakamura T. Neuroprotection and enhanced recovery with edaravone after acute spinal cord injury in rats. Spine (Phila Pa 1976). 2005;**30**:1154-1158

[20] Pannu R, Barbosa E, Singh AK, Singh I. Attenuation of acute inflammatory response by atorvastatin after spinal cord injury in rats. Journal of Neuroscience Research. 2005;**79**: 340-350. DOI: 10.1002/jnr.20345

[21] Arataki S, Tomizawa K, Moriwaki A, Nishida K, Matsushita M, Ozaki T, et al. Calpain inhibitors prevent neuronal cell death and ameliorate motor disturbances after compression-induced spinal cord injury in rats. Journal of Neurotrauma. 2005;**22**: 398-406. DOI: 10.1089/neu.2005.22.398

[22] Ahmad M, Zakaria A, Almutairi KM. Effectiveness of minocycline and FK506 alone and in combination on enhanced behavioral and biochemical recovery from spinal cord injury in rats. Pharmacology, Biochemistry, and Behavior. 2016;**145**:45-54. DOI: 10.1016/j.pbb.2016.04.003

[23] Yao M, Yang L, Wang J, Sun YL, Dun RL, Wang YJ, et al. Neurological recovery and antioxidant effects of curcumin for spinal cord injury in the rat: A network meta-analysis and systematic review. Journal of Neurotrauma. 2015;**32**:381-391. DOI: 10.1089/neu.2014.3520

[24] Yang L, Yao M, Lan Y, Mo W, Sun YL, Wang J, et al. Melatonin for spinal cord injury in animal models: A systematic review and network meta-analysis. Journal of Neurotrauma. 2016;**33**:290-300. DOI: 10.1089/neu.2015.4038

[25] Yong VW, Wells J, Giullani F, Casha S, Power C, Metz LM. The promise of minocycline in neurology. Lancet Neurology. 2004;**3**:744-751. DOI: 10.1016/S1474-4422(04)00937-8

[26] Kim HS, Suh YH. Minocycline and neurodegenerative diseases. Behavioural Brain Research. 2009;**196**:168-179. DOI: 10.1016/j.bbr.2008.09.040

[27] Garrido-Mesa N, Zarzuelo A, Galvez J. Minocycline: Far beyond an antibiotic. British Journal of Pharmacology. 2013;**169**:337-352. DOI: 10.1111/bph.12139

[28] Wang Z, Nong J, Shultz RB, Zhang Z, Kim T, Tom VJ, et al. Local delivery of minocycline from metal ion-assisted self-assembled complexes promotes neuroprotection and functional recovery after spinal cord injury. Biomaterials. 2017;**112**:62-71. DOI: 10.1016/j.biomaterials.2016.10.002

[29] Plane JM, Shen Y, Pleasure DE, Deng W. Prospects for minocycline neuroprotection. Archives of Neurology.

2010;**67**:1442-1448. DOI: 10.1001/archneurol.2010.191

[30] Ghazali H, Wu W, Abdullah MA. Histological analysis of motoneuron survival and microglia inhibition after nerve root avulsion treated with nerve graft implantation and minocycline: An experimental study. Sains Malaysiana. 2016;**45**:1641-1648

[31] Chin TY, Kiat SS, Faizul HG, Wu W, Abdullah JM. The effects of minocycline on spinal root avulsion injury in rat model. Malaysian Journal of Medical Sciences. 2017;**24**:31-39. DOI: 10.21315/mjms2017.24.1.4

[32] Garcia-Martinez EM, Sanz-Blasco S, Karachitos A, Bandez MJ, Fernandez-Gomez FJ, Prez-Alvarez S, et al. Mitochondria and calcium flux as targets of neuroprotection caused by minocycline in cerebellar granule cells. Biochemical Pharmacology. 2010;**79**:239-250. DOI: 10.1016/j.bcp.2009.07.028

[33] Takeda M, Kawaguchi M, Kumatoriya T, Horiuchi T, Watanabe K, Inoue S, et al. Effects of minocycline on hind-limb motor function and gray and white matter injury after spinal cord ischemia in rats. Spine (Phila Pa 1976). 2011;**36**:1919-1924. DOI: 10.1097/BRS.0b013e3181ffda29

[34] Yune TY, Lee JY, Jung GY, Kim SJ, Jiang MH, Kim YC, et al. Minocycline alleviates death of oligodendrocytes by inhibiting pro-nerve growth factor production in microglia after spinal cord injury. The Journal of Neuroscience. 2007;**27**:7751-7761. DOI: 10.1523/JNEUROSCI.1661-07.2007

[35] Ma L, Nagai J, Ueda H. Microglial activation mediates de novo lysophosphatidic acid production in a model of neuropathic pain. Journal of Neurochemistry. 2010;**115**:643-653. DOI: 10.1111/j.1471-4159.2010.06955.x

[36] Pang T, Wang J, Benicky J, Saavedra JM. Minocycline ameliorates LPS-induced inflammation in human monocytes by novel mechanisms including LOX-1, Nur77 and LITAF inhibition. Biochimica et Biophysica Acta. 1820;**2012**:503-510. DOI: 10.1016/j.bbagen.2012.01.011

[37] Chu LS, Fang SH, Zhou Y, Yin YJ, Chen WY, Li JH, et al. Minocycline inhibits 5-lipoxygenase expression and accelerates functional recovery in chronic phase of focal cerebral ischemia in rats. Life Sciences. 2010;**86**:170-177. DOI: 10.1016/j.lfs.2009.12.001

[38] Shultz RB, Zhong YZ. Minocycline targets multiple secondary injury mechanisms in traumatic spinal cord injury. Neural Regeneration Research. 2017;**12**:702-713. DOI: 10.4103/1673-5374.206633

[39] Sonmez E, Kabatas S, Ozen O, Karabey G, Turkoglu S, Ogus E, et al. Minocycline treatment inhibits lipid peroxidation, preserves spinal cord ultrastructure, and improves functional outcome after traumatic spinal cord injury in the rat. Spine (Phila Pa 1976). 2013;**38**:1253-1259. DOI: 10.1097/BRS.0b013e3182895587

[40] Aras M, Altas M, Motor S, Dokuyucu R, Yilmaz A, Ozgiray E, et al. Protective effects of minocycline on experimental spinal cord injury in rats. Injury. 2015;**46**:1471-1474. DOI: 10.1016/j.injury.2015.05.018

[41] Zhang H, Chang M, Hansen CN, Basso DM, Noble-Haeusslein LJ. Role of matrix metalloproteinases and therapeutic benefits of their inhibition in spinal cord injury. Neurotherapeutics. 2011;**8**:206-220. DOI: 10.1007/s13311-011-0038-0

[42] Modheji M, Olapour S, Khodaya MJ, Jalili A, Yaghooti H. Minocycline is more potent than tetracycline and doxycline in inhibiting MMP-9

in vitro. Jundishapur Journal of Natural Pharmaceutical Products. 2016;**11**:e273377

[43] Lee S, Yune TY, Kim SI, Paark W, Lee YK, Km YC, et al. Minocycline reduces cell death and improves functional recovery after traumatic spinal cord injury in the rat. Journal of Neurotrauma. 2003;**10**:1017-1027. DOI: 10.1089/089771503770195867

[44] Stirling DP, Khodarahmi K, Liu J, McPhail LT, McBride CB, Steeves JD, et al. Minocycline treatment reduces delayed oligodendrocyte death, attenuates axonal dieback, and improves functional outcome after spinal cord injury. The Journal of Neuroscience. 2004;**24**:2182-2190. DOI: 10.1523/JNEUROSCI.5275-03.2004

[45] Wells JE, Hurlbert RJ, Fehlings MG, Yong VW. Neuroprotection by minocycline facilitates significant recovery from spinal cord injury in mice. Brain. 2003;**126**:1628-1637. DOI: 10.1093/brain/awg178

[46] Squair JW, Ruiz I, Phillips AA, Zheng MMZ, Sarafis ZK, Sachdeva R, et al. Minocycline reduces the severity of autonomic dysreflexia after experimental spinal cord injury. Journal of Neurotrauma. 2018;**35**:2861-2871. DOI: 10.1089/neu.2018.5703

[47] Saganova K, Orendacova J, Cizkova D, Vanickv I. Limited minocycline neuroprotection after balloon-compression spinal cord injury in the rat. Neuroscience Letters. 2008;**433**:246-249. DOI: 10.1016/j.neulet.2008.01.041

[48] Cho DC, Cheong JH, Yang MS, Hwang SJ, Kim JM, Kim CH. The effect of minocycline on motor neuron recovery and neuropathic pain in a rat model of spinal cord injury. Journal of Korean Neurosurgical Association. 2011;**49**:83-91. DOI: 10.3340/jkns.2011.49.2.83

[49] Su Z, Yuan Y, Cao L, Zhu Y, Gao L, Qiu Y, et al. Triptolide promotes spinal cord repair by inhibiting astrogliosis and inflammation. Glia. 2010;**58**:901-915. DOI: 10.1002/glia.20972

[50] Drenger B, Blanck TJJ, Jaffery BPE, Recino-Pinto E, Sideris A. Minocycline before aortic occlusion reduces hindlimb motor impairment, attenuates spinal cord damage and spinal astrocytosis, and preserve neural cytoarchitecture in the rat. Journal of Cardiothoracic and Vascular Anesthesia. 2019;**33**:1003-1011. DOI: 10.1053/j. jvca.2018.07.028

[51] Chen D, Zeng W, Fu Y, Gao M, Lv G. Bone marrow mesenchymal stem cells combined with minocycline improve spinal cord injury in a rat model. International Journal of Clinical and Experimental Pathology. 2015;**8**:11957-11969

[52] Ibarra A, Hernandez E, Lomeli J, Pineda D, Buenrostro M, Martinon S, et al. MadrazoI: Cyclosporin-A enhances non-functional axonal growing after complete spinal cord transaction. Brain Research. 2007;**1149**:200-209. DOI: 10.1016/j.brainres.2007.02.056

[53] Chen ZR, Ma Y, Guo HH, Lu ZD, Jin QH. Therapeutic efficacy of cyclosporin a against spinal cord injury in rats with hyperglycemia. Molecular Medicine Reports. 2018;**17**:4369-4375. DOI: 10.3892/mmr.2018.8422

[54] Gao SJ, Liu Y, Wang HJ, Ban DX, Cheng SZ, Ning GZ, et al. New approach to treating spinal cord injury using PEG-TAT-modified, cyclosporine-A-loaded PLGA/polymeric liposomes. Journal of Drug Targeting. 2017;**25**:75-82. DOI: 10.1080/1061186X.2016.1191082

[55] Ibarra A, Diaz-Ruiz A. Protective effect of cyclosporin-A in spinal cord injury: An overview. Current Medicinal Chemistry. 2006;**13**:2703-2710

[56] Diaz-Ruiz A, Vergara P, Perez-Severiano F, Segovia J, Guizar-Sahagun G, Ibarra A, et al. Cyclosporin-A inhibits constitutive nitric oxide synthase activity and neuronal and endothelial nitric oxide synthase expressions after spinal cord injury in rats. Neurochemical Research. 2005;**30**:245-251

[57] Gold BG. Neuroimmunophillin ligands: Evaluation of their therapeutic potential for the treatment of neurological disorders. Expert Opinion on Investigational Drugs. 2000;**9**:2331-2342. DOI: 10.1517/13543784.9.10.2331

[58] Roozbehi A, Joghataie MT, Mehdizadeh M, Mirzaei A, Delaviz H. The effects of cyclosporine-A on functional outcome and axonal regrowth following spinal cord injury in adult rats. Acta Medica Iranica. 2012;**50**:226-232

[59] Ibarra A, Correa D, Willms K, Merchant MT, Guizar-Sahagun G, Grijalva I, et al. Effects of cyclosporin-A on immune response, tissue protection and motor function of rats subjected to spinal cord injury. Brain Research. 2003;**979**:165-178

[60] Yousuf S, Atif F, Kesharwani V, Agrawal SK. Neuroprotective effects of Tacrolimus (FK-506) and Cyclosporin (CsA) in oxidative injury. Brain and Behavior: A Cognitive Neuroscience Perspective. 2011;**1**:87-94. DOI: 10.1002/brb3.16

[61] Khankan RR, Griffis KG, Haggerty-Skeans JR, Zhong H, Roy RR, Edgerton VR, et al. Olfactory ensheathing cell transplantation after a complete spinal cord transection mediates neuroprotective and immunomodulatory mechanisms to facilitate regeneration. The Journal of Neuroscience. 2016;**36**:6269-6286. DOI: 10.1523/JNEUROSCI.0085-16.2016

[62] Starzl TE, Todo S, Fung J, Demetris AJ, Venkataramman R, Jain A. FK506 for liver, kidney and pancreas transplantation. Lancet. 1989;**2**:1000-1004

[63] Sosa I, Reyes O, Kuffler DP. Immunosuppressants: Neuroprotection and promoting neurological recovery following peripheral nerve and spinal cord lesions. Experimental Neurology. 2005;**195**:7-15. DOI: 10.1016/j.expneurol.2005.04.016

[64] Bochelen DMR, Sauter A. Calcineurin inhibitors FK506 and SDZASM981 alleviate the outcome of focal cerebral ischemic/reperfusion injury. The Journal of Pharmacology and Experimental Therapeutics. 1999;**288**:653-659

[65] Butcher SP, Henshall DC, Teramura Y, Iwasaki K, Sharkey J. Neuroprotective actions of FK506 in experimental stroke: In vivo evidence against an antiexcitotoxic mechanism. The Journal of Neuroscience. 1997;**17**:6939-6946

[66] Madsen JR, McDonald P, Irwin N, Goldberg DE, Yao GL, Meiri KF, et al. Tacrolimus (FK506) increases neuronal expression of GAP-43 and improves functional recovery after spinal cord injury in rats. Experimental Neurology. 1998;**154**:673-683. DOI: 10.1006/exnr.1998.6974

[67] Saganova K, Galik J, Blasko J, Korimova A, Racekova E, Vanicky I. Immunosuppressant FK506: Focusing on neuroprotective effects following brain and spinal cord injury. Life Sciences. 2012;**91**:77-82. DOI: 10.1016/j.lfs.2012.06.022

[68] Pan F, Chen A, Guo F, Zhu C, Tao F. Effect of FK506 on expression of hepatocyte growth factor in murine spinal cord following peripheral nerve injury. Journal of Huazhong University of Science and Technology. Medical

Sciences. 2008;**28**:159-162. DOI: 10.1007/s11596-008-0211-9

[69] Yamaji T, Yamazaki S, Li J, Price RD, Matsuoka N, Mutoh S. FK1706, a novel non-immunosuppressant neurophilin ligand, ameliorates motor dysfunction following spinal cord injury through its neurodegenerative action. European Journal of Pharmacology. 2008;**591**:147-152. DOI: 10.1016/j.ejphar.2008.06.064

[70] Gordon T, Sulaiman O, Boyd JG. Experimental strategies to promote functional recovery after peripheral nerve injuries. Journal of the Peripheral Nervous System. 2003;**8**:236-250

[71] Navarro X, Udina E, Ceballos D, Gold BG. Effects of FK506 on nerve regeneration and re innervation after graft or tube repair of long nerve gaps. Muscle & Nerve. 2001;**24**:905-915

[72] Sulaiman OA, Voda J, Gold BG, Gordon T. FK506 increases peripheral nerve regeneration after chronic axotomy but not after chronic Schwann cell denervation. Experimental Neurology. 2002;**175**:127-137. DOI: 10.1006/exnr.2002.7878

[73] Udina E, Rodrigues FJ, Verdu E, Espejo M, Gold BG, Navarro X. FK506 enhances regeneration of axons across long peripheral nerve gaps repaired with collagen guides seeded with allogenic Schwann cells. Glia. 2004;**47**:120-129. DOI: 10.1002/glia.20025

[74] Cai J, Sun Y, Yin Z, Wang D, Shi K, Fu Y, et al. Analysis of FK506-mediated functional recovery and neuroprotection in a rat model of spinal cord injury indicates that EGF is modulated in astrocytes. Experimental and Therapeutic Medicine. 2018;**16**: 501-510. DOI: 10.3892/etm.2018.6283

[75] Devaux S, Cizkoya D, Mallah K, Karnoub MA, Laouby Z, Kobeissv F, et al. RhoA inhibitor treatment at acute phase of spinal cord injury may induce neurite outgrowth and synaptogenesis. Molecular & Cellular Proteomics. 2017;**16**:1394-1415. DOI: 10.1074/mcp.M116.064881

[76] Chen G, Zhang Z, Wang S, Lv D. Combined treatment with FK506 and nerve growth factor for spinal cord injury in rats. Experimental and Therapeutic Medicine. 2013;**6**:868-872. DOI: 10.3892/etm.2013.1254

[77] Kaymaz M, Emmez H, Bukan N, Dursun A, Kurt G, Pasaoglu A. Effectiveness of FK506 on lipid peroxidation in the spinal cord following experimental traumatic injury. Spinal Cord. 2005;**43**:22-26. DOI: 10.1038/sj.sc.3101621

[78] Sharif-Alhoseini M, Rahimi-Movaghar V. Animal models in traumatic spinal cord injury. In: Dionyssiotis Y, editor. Topics in Paraplegia. UK: Intechopen Limited; 2014. pp. 209-228. DOI: 10.5772/57189

[79] Zhang N, Fang M, Chen H, Gou F, Ding M. Evaluation of spinal cord injury animal models. Neural Regeneration Research. 2014;**9**:2008-2012. DOI: 10.4103/1673-5374.143436

[80] Lee DH, Lee JK. Animal models of axon regeneration after spinal cord injury. Neuroscience Bulletin. 2013;**29**:436-444. DOI: 10.1007/s12264-013-1365-4

[81] Koozekanani SH, Vise WM, Hashemi RM, McGhee RB. Possible mechanisms for observed pathophysiological variability in experimental spinal cord injury by the method of Allen. Journal of Neurosurgery. 1976;**44**:429-434

[82] Piao MS, Lee JK, Jang JW, Kim SH, Kim HS. A mouse model of photochemically induced spinal cord injury. Journal of Korean Neurosurgical Association. 2009;**46**:479-483. DOI: 10.3340/jkns.2009.46.5.479

[83] Min SH, Lee SH, Shim H, Park JS, Lee YI, Kim HW, et al. Development of complete thoracic spinal cord transection model in rats for delayed transplantation of stem cells. Spine (Phila Pa 1976). 2011;**36**:155-163. DOI: 10.1097/BRS.0b013e3181d8b92a

[84] Seifert JL, Bell JE, Elmer BB, Sucato DJ, Romero MI. Characterization of a novel bidirectional distraction spinal cord injury animal model. Journal of Neuroscience Methods. 2011;**197**:97-103. DOI: 10.1016/j.jneumeth.2011.02.003

[85] Lacifi G, Gedik HS, Korkmaz K, Erdem H, Cicek OF, Nacar OA, et al. Efficacy of iloprost and montelukast combination on spinal cord ischemia/reperfusion injury in a rat model. Journal of Cardiothoracic Surgery. 2013;**4**:8-64. DOI: 10.1186/1749-8090-8-64

[86] Yeo SJ, Hwang SN, Park SW, Kim YB, Min BK, Kwon JT, et al. Development of a rat model of graded contusive spinal cord injury using a pneumatic impact device. Journal of Korean Medical Science. 2004;**19**:574-580. DOI: 10.3346/jkms.2004.19.4.574

[87] Vijayaprakash KM, Sridharan N. An experimental spinal cord injury rat model using customized impact device: A cost-effective approach. Journal of Pharmacology and Pharmacotherapeutics. 2013;**4**:211-213. DOI: 10.4103/0976-500X.114607

[88] Blight AR. Morphometric analysis of a model of spinal cord injury in Guinea pigs, with behavioral evidence of delayed secondary pathology. Journal of the Neurological Sciences. 1991;**103**:156-171

[89] Nystrom B, Berglund JE. Spinal cord restitution following compression injuries in rats. Acta Neurologica Scandinavica. 1998;**78**:467-472

[90] Van Meeteren NL, Eggers R, Lankhorst AJ, Gispen WH, Hamers FP. Locomotor recovery after spinal cord contusion injury in rats is improved by spontaneous exercise. Journal of Neurotrauma. 2003;**20**:1029-1037. DOI: 10.4103/1673-5374.143436

[91] Zeman RJ, Wen X, Ouyang N, Rocchio R, Shih L, Alfieri A, et al. Stereotactic radiosurgery improves locomotor recovery after spinal cord injury in rats. Neurosurgery. 2008;**63**:981-987. DOI: 10.1227/01.NEU.0000330404.37092.3E

[92] Lee JH, Tigchelaar S, Liu J, Stammers AM, Streijger F, Tetzlaff W, et al. Lack of neuroprotective effects of simvastatin and minocycline in a model of cervical spinal cord injury. Experimental Neurology. 2010;**225**:219-230. DOI: 10.1016/j.expneurol.2010.06.018

[93] McMahon SS, Albermann S, Rooney GE, Moran C, Hynes J, Garcia Y, et al. Effect of cyclosporin A on functional recovery in the spinal cord following contusion injury. Journal of Anatomy. 2009;**215**:267-279. DOI: 10.1111/j.1469-7580.2009.01107.x

[94] Basso DM, Beattie MS, Bresnahan JC. A sensitive and reliable locomotor rating scale for open field testing in rats. Journal of Neurotrauma. 1995;**12**:1-21. DOI: 10.1089/neu.1995.12

[95] Tarlov IM, Klinger H. Spinal cord compression studies. AMA Archives of Neurology and Psychiatry. 1954;**71**:275-290

[96] Rivlin AS, Tator CH. Objective clinical assessment of motor function after experimental spinal cord injury in the rat. Journal of Neurosurgery. 1977;**47**:577-581

[97] Gale K, Kerasidis H, Wrathall JR. Spinal cord contusion in the rat: Behavioral analysis of functional neurologic impairment. Experimental Neurology. 1985;**88**:123-134

[98] Kerasidis H, Wrathall JR, Gale K. Behavioral assessment of functional deficit in rats with contusive spinal cord injury. Journal of Neuroscience Methods. 1987;**20**:167-179

[99] Patrick OE, Hirohisa M, Masahira K, Koreaki M. Central nervous system bioaminergic responses to mechanic trauma. Surgical Neurology. 1991;**35**:273-279

[100] Ohkawa H, Ohishi N, Yagi K. Assay for lipid peroxides in animal tissues by thiobarbituric acid reaction. Analytical Biochemistry. 1979;**95**:351-358

[101] Jo C, Ahn DU. Fluorometric analysis of 2-thiobarbituric acid reactive substances. Poultry Science. 1998;**77**:475-480. DOI: 10.1093/ps/77.3.475

[102] Mangino MJ, Murphy MK, Glabar GG, Anderson CB. Protective effects of glycine perfusion injury. The American Journal of Physiology. 1991;**261**:F841-F848. DOI: 10.1152/ajprenal.1991.261.5.F841

[103] Tariq M, Morais C, Kishore PN, Biary N, Al Deeb S, Al Moutaery K. Neurological recovery in diabetic rats following spinal cord injury. Journal of Neurotrauma. 1998;**15**:239-251. DOI: 10.1089/neu.1998.15.239

[104] Bradley PP, Priebat DA, Christensen RD, Rothstein G. Measurement of cutaneous inflammation: Estimation of neutrophil content with an enzyme marker. The Journal of Investigative Dermatology. 1982;**78**:206-209

[105] Dumont RJ, Okonkwo DO, Verma S, Hurlbert RJ, Boulos PT, Ellegala DB, et al. Acute spinal cord injury, part I: Pathophysiologic mechanisms. Clinical Neuropharmacology. 2001;**24**:254-264

[106] Kaptanoglu E, Tuncel M, Palaoglu S, Konan A, Demirpence E, Kilinc K. Comparison of the effects of melatonin and methylprednisolone in experimental spinal cord injury. Journal of Neurosurgery. 2000;**93**:77-84

[107] Antri M, Orsal D, Barthe JY. Locomotor recovery in the chronic spinal rat: Effects of long-term treatment with a 5-HT2 agonist. The European Journal of Neuroscience. 2002;**6**:467-476

[108] Zhang J, Zhang A, Sun Y, Cao X, Zhang N. Treatment with immunosuppressants FTY720 and tacrolimus promotes functional recovery after spinal cord injury in rats. The Tohoku Journal of Experimental Medicine. 2009;**219**:295-302

[109] Vafadari R, Kraaijeveld R, Weimar W, Baan CC. Tacrolimus inhibits NF-κB activation in peripheral human T cells. PLoS One. 2013;**8**:e60784. DOI: 10.1371/journal.pone.0060784

[110] Romero SE, Bravo G, Hong E, Rojas G, Ibarra A. Acute, subacute and chronic effect of cyclosporin-A on mean arterial pressure of rats with severe spinal cord contusion. Neuroscience Letters. 2008;**445**:99-102. DOI: 10.1016/j.neulet.2008.08.063

[111] Zhou YQ, Liu DQ, Chen SP, Sun J, Wang XM, Tian YK, et al. Minocycline as a promising therapeutic strategy for chronic pain. Pharmacological Research. 2018;**134**:305-310. DOI: 10.1016/j.phrs.2018.07.002

[112] Noga BR, Pinzon A, Mesigil RP, Hentall ID. Steady-state levels of monoamines in the rat lumbar spinal cord: Spatial mapping and the effect of acute spinal cord injury. Journal of Neurophysiology. 2004;**92**:567-577. DOI: 10.1152/jn.01035.2003

[113] Bravo G, Ibarra A, Guizar-Sahagun G, Rojas G, Hong E. Indorenate improves motor function in rats with chronic spinal cord injury.

Basic & Clinical Pharmacology & Toxicology. 2007;**100**:67-70. DOI: 10.1111/j.172-7843.2007.00004.x

[114] Taoka Y, Okajima K, Uchiba M, Murakami K, Kushimoto S, Johno M, et al. Role of neutrophils in spinal cord injury in rats. Neuroscience. 1997;**79**:1177-1182

[115] Genovese T, Mazzon E, Di Paola R, Cannavo G, Muia C, Bramanti P, et al. Role of endogenous ligands for the peroxisome proliferators activated receptors alpha in the secondary damage in experimental spinal cord trauma. Experimental Neurology. 2005;**194**:267-278. DOI: 10.1016/j.expneurol.2005.03.003

[116] Voda J, Hama A, Sagen J. FK506 reduces the severity of cutaneous hypersensitivity in rats with a spinal cord contusion. Neuroscience Research. 2007;**58**:95-99. DOI: 10.1016/j.neures.2007.02.004

[117] Kwon BK, Tetzlaff W, Grauer JN, Beiner J, Vaccaro AR. Pathophysiology and pharmacologic treatment of acute spinal cord injury. The Spine Journal. 2004;**4**:451-464. DOI: 10.1016/j.spinee.2003.07.007

[118] Lee VM, Hartley RS, Trojanowski JQ. Neurobiology of human neurons (NT2N) grafted into mouse spinal cord: Implications for improving therapy of spinal cord injury. Progress in Brain Research. 2000;**128**:299-307. DOI: 10.1016/S0079-6123(00)28027-8

[119] Anthes DL, Theriault E, Tator CH. Ultrastructural evidence for arteriolar vasospasm after spinal cord trauma. Neurosurgery. 1996;**39**:804-814

[120] Blight AR. Cellular morphology of chronic spinal cord injury in the cat: Analysis of myelinated axons by line-sampling. Neuroscience. 1983;**10**:521-543

[121] Beattie MS, Li Q, Bresnahan JC. Cell death and plasticity after experimental spinal cord injury. Progress in Brain Research. 2000;**128**:9-21. DOI: 10.1016/S0079-6123(00)28003-5

[122] Kakulas BA. A review the neuropathology of human spinal cord injury with emphasis on special features. The Journal of Spinal Cord Medicine. 1999;**22**:119-124

[123] Iwasa K, Ikata T, Fukuzawa K. Protective effect of vitamin E on spinal cord injury by compression and concurrent lipid peroxidation. Free Radical Biology & Medicine. 1989;**6**:599-606

[124] Agrawal SK, Fehlings MG. The effect of the sodium channel blocker QX-314 on recovery after acute spinal cord injury. Journal of Neurotrauma. 1997;**14**:81-88. DOI: 10.1089/neu.1997.14.81

[125] Springer JE, Azbill RD, Knapp PE. Activation of the caspase-3 apoptic cascade in traumatic spinal cord injury. Nature Medicine. 1999;**5**:943-946. DOI: 10.1038/11387

[126] Citron BA, Smirnova IV, Arnold PM, Festoff BW. Upregulation of neurotoxic serine proteases, prothrombin, and protease-activated receptor 1 early after spinal cord injury. Journal of Neurotrauma. 2000;**17**:1191-1203. DOI: 101089/neu.2000.17.1191

[127] Stys PK, Waxman SG, Ransom BR. Ionic mechanisms of anoxic injury in mammalian CNS white matter: Role of Na+ channels and Na(+)-Ca2+ exchanger. The Journal of Neuroscience. 1992;**12**:430-439

[128] Crowe MJ, Bresnahan JC, Shuman SL, Masters JN, Beattie MS. Apoptosis and delayed degeneration after spinal cord injury in rats and monkeys. Nature Medicine. 1997;**73**:73-76

[129] Liu XZ, Xu XM, Hu R, Du C, Zhang SX, McDonald JW, et al. Neuronal and glial apoptosis after traumatic spinal cord injury. The Journal of Neuroscience. 1997;**17**:5395-5406

[130] Hall ED, Wolf DL. A pharmacological analysis of the pathophysiological mechanisms of posttraumatic spinal cord ischemia. Journal of Neurosurgery. 1986;**64**:951-961. DOI: 10.3171/jns.1986.64.6.0951

[131] Young W, Koreh I. Potassium and calcium changes in injured spinal cord. Brain Research. 1986;**365**:42-53

[132] Plant GW, Christensen CL, Oudega M, Bunge MB. Delayed transplantation of olfactory ensheathing glia promotes sparing/regeneration of supraspinal axons in the contused adult rat spinal cord. Journal of Neurotrauma. 2003;**20**:1-16. DOI: 10.1089/08977150360517146

[133] Verdu E, Garcia-Alias G, Fores J, Lopez-Vales R, Navarro X. Olfactory ensheathing cells transplanted in lesioned spinal cord prevent loss of spinal cord parenchyma and promote functional recovery. Glia. 2003;**42**: 275-286. DOI: 10.1002/glia.10217

[134] Ahmad M, Abo Shaiqah A, Alshehri AS, Alotaibi AM. Accentuated rehabilitation recovery from spinal cord injury in rats through increased behavioral activity besides minocycline treatment: A nursing care perspective. JOJ Nurse Health Care. 2018;**5**:555674. DOI: 10.19080/JOJNHC.2018.05.555674

Section 3

Non-Pharmacological Therapies

Chapter 6

Noninvasive Modalities Used in Spinal Cord Injury Rehabilitation

Filipe O. Barroso, Alejandro Pascual-Valdunciel, Diego Torricelli, Juan C. Moreno, Antonio Del Ama-Espinosa, Jozsef Laczko and José L. Pons

Abstract

In the past three decades, research on plasticity after spinal cord injury (SCI) has led to a gradual shift in SCI rehabilitation: the former focus on learning compensatory strategies changed to functional neurorecovery, that is, promoting restoration of function through the use of affected limbs. This paradigm shift contributed to the development of technology-based interventions aiming to promote neurorecovery through repetitive training. This chapter presents an overview of a range of noninvasive modalities that have been used in rehabilitation after SCI. Among others, we present repetitive transcranial magnetic stimulation (rTMS), transcranial direct current stimulation (tDCS), surface electrical stimulation tools such as transcutaneous electrical spinal cord stimulation (tcSCS), transcutaneous electrical nerve stimulation (TENS), and functional electrical stimulation (FES), as well as its integration with cycling training and assistive robotic devices. The most recent results attained and the potential relevance of these new techniques to strengthen the efficacy of the residual neuronal pathways and improve spasticity are also presented. Future efforts toward the widespread clinical application of these modalities include more advances in the technology, together with the knowledge obtained from basic research and clinical trials. This can ultimately lead to novel customized interventions that meet specific needs of SCI patients.

Keywords: spinal cord injury, rehabilitation, noninvasive modalities, functional electrical stimulation, transcranial magnetic stimulation, exoskeletons

1. Introduction

Spinal cord injury (SCI) is an event that affects the quality of life of patients as a consequence of affected sexual function, impaired sensory and motor function, including bowel and bladder control, walking, eating, grasping, pain, and spasticity [1–3]. For many years, SCI has been considered irreversible [4]. However, research on plasticity after SCI has opened new paths and generated a shift in rehabilitation of SCI patients in the past three decades: its former focus on learning compensatory movements to regain function gradually changed to restoration of function through repetitive movement training combined with the stimulation of the nervous system [5].

IntechOpen

The term neural plasticity describes the ability of the nervous system to adapt a new functional or structural state in response to intrinsic or extrinsic factors [6]. Thus, plasticity encompasses the underlying mechanisms that lead to a spontaneous return or recover of motor, sensory and autonomic functions to different degrees. The concept of plasticity at the cellular level can be tracked back to Ramon y Cajal's work, who suggested that modification of synaptic connections could play a very important role in memory [7]. After that, the work of Donald Hebb was very important to the concept of long-term potentiation (LTP), namely by suggesting that two neurons that fire together and are close enough may grow some connections or undergo metabolic changes that increase their ability to communicate [8]. This happens because chemical synapses have the ability to change their strength [9].

Sensory information from Ia afferent fibers (transmitting information about muscle activity and movement) play an essential role in inducing functional and morphological changes that lead to the maturation of the brain and the spinal cord [9], independently of the SCI level and whether it is complete or incomplete [10]. Thus, activity-dependent plasticity refers to the changes in the central nervous system (CNS) associated with movement [9] and reflects one of the basic forms of learning in humans [11]. These neural changes happen throughout the life span at both the brain and spinal cord level. However, not all plasticity is beneficial: adverse changes may also appear [12]. This is known as maladaptive plasticity and encompasses events such as excessive plasticity associated with some disease symptoms like focal dystonia, spasticity, and chronic pain. Current SCI rehabilitation is based on task-specific programs aiming at promoting neurorecovery through beneficial activity-dependent plasticity and avoiding maladaptive plasticity [6].

This chapter summarizes the main effects on motor and functional recovery, as well as spasticity and pain, when using noninvasive modalities in the rehabilitation of SCI patients, either in the research or the clinical setting. Some of these techniques aim at stimulating different levels of the central (brain or spinal cord) and peripheral nervous system, while others combine some sort of stimulation with devices that may assist and allow for repetitive motor training (e.g., hybrid exoskeletons and FES driven cycling).

2. Brain stimulation

Recent research has shown that even complete SCI patients may preserve some residual pathways connecting supraspinal and spinal circuits [13]. Given that these patients may preserve muscle activity below the level of injury, target rehabilitation for SCI also includes modalities that stimulate the brain. This might strengthen the efficacy of the residual neural pathways and, therefore, improve volitional control after SCI [14]. This section describes two different types of noninvasive brain stimulation (NIBS): repetitive transcranial magnetic stimulation (rTMS) and transcranial direct current stimulation (tDCS). Both techniques have been used in the research and clinical setting aiming at improving motor and functional recovery, as well as spasticity and pain after SCI [4].

2.1 Repetitive transcranial magnetic stimulation (rTMS)

Transcranial magnetic stimulation (TMS) is a form of noninvasive brain stimulation in which short magnetic fields are generated by a coil in order to induce electric current pulses in the brain, which can then elicit depolarization and action potentials in cortical neurons (see **Figure 1**). Since its first application in humans in 1985, TMS has become a standard electrophysiological technique to

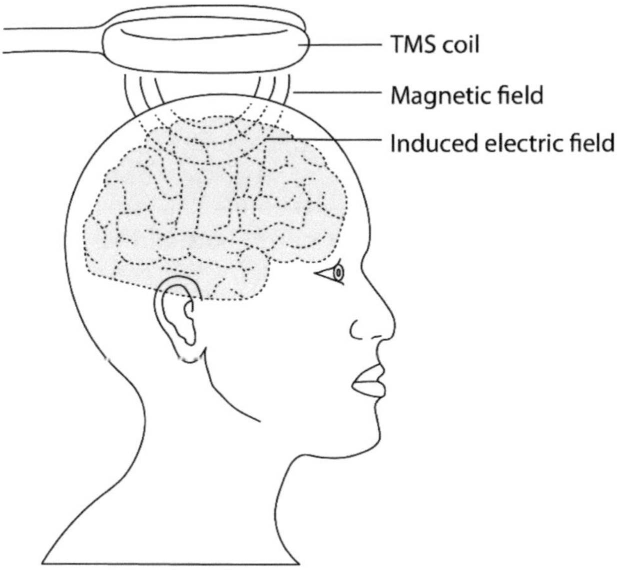

Figure 1.
The magnetic field generated by the TMS coil will induce electric current pulses in the brain, which can elicit depolarization and action potentials in cortical neurons.

assess the excitability of the corticospinal circuitry, due to its usability and ability to directly activate brain structures without causing harm to the subject. The most extended protocol applies single TMS pulses to activate motor cortex at a specific area where topographic projections of a group of muscles are represented. This cortical activation elicits action potentials that propagate until reaching the muscles, inducing a motor evoked potential (MEP), which can be measured by electromyography (EMG) [2].

Repetitive transcranial magnetic stimulation (rTMS) is a form of TMS where several TMS pulses are applied sequentially in order to induce long-term changes in the targeted neural pathways. The underlying physiological mechanism of rTMS lies in the repeated activation of a network of synapses that may lead to long-term potentiation (LTP) or long-term depression (LTD) of those synapses [4]. The induction of long-term changes in neural circuits using rTMS can be applied to revert the effects of neurological disorders. For instance, rTMS received FDA approval and has become a promising treatment for major depression.

Due to its ability to induce long-term changes in neural systems, rTMS has been also applied in patients with motor disorders as a modality to modulate the activity of residual (cortical, subcortical, and corticospinal) pathways and thus promote functional recovery [2]. Moreover, rTMS has been applied in a wide range of protocols, with varying frequencies and intensities of stimulation, or even the number of pulses and sessions, among others. The main stimulation protocols explored so far may be encompassed in the following:

- Theta burst stimulation (TBS) consists of three 50 Hz pulses delivered in blocks at 200-ms interval (5 Hz). Intermittent TBS (iTBS) involves the delivery of TBS for 2 s, followed by a resting period of 8 seconds, for a total of 3 min; this is hypothesized to facilitate LTP [15]. On the other hand, continuous TBS (cTBS) applied in 40 s blocks promote LTD.

- QuadroPulse (qQPS) applies four high-frequency pulses repeated every 5 s. The facilitator or inhibitory excitability effects depend on the inter-pulse intervals.

- I-wave protocol involves the repetitive stimulation of the motor cortex at 1.5 ms rate, seeking to mimic the indirect waves (I-waves) of corticospinal neurons and to increase their excitability [4].

- Paired associative stimulation (PAS) relies on the Hebb's theory, which states that a synaptic connection is enhanced when two stimuli converge in time repeatedly. PAS protocol combines a peripheral nerve stimulus with a TMS pulse over the motor cortex, aiming to pair both stimuli in time at the cortex, which will promote corticospinal excitability. PAS can present different variants, in which the TMS pulse can be replaced by physiological activation of the motor cortex (e.g., imaginary movement), or the pairing site targets of TMS and peripheral stimulus are the motoneurons at the spinal cord.

Regardless of its incipient stage and current limitations, rTMS has become a promising approach for SCI rehabilitation, not only to improve motor function but also to decrease spasticity and neuropathic pain. This technique enables targeting and promoting long-term changes in neural pathways, by exploiting the plastic properties that may facilitate function recovery. Improvements seem to be present when higher rTMS stimulus intensities are used [2]. On the other hand, the few studies that investigated the effects of rTMS on spasticity in iSCI patients reported some reduction in the clinical symptoms of spasticity [2]. Moreover, the few studies that tested the effect of rTMS on neuropathic pain reported some reductions in the clinical symptoms of pain [2].

Notwithstanding, these results hold a great variability, are not reproducible in all patients, and are limited to certain clinical assessment scales or neurophysiological measurements. Several constraints can explain current limitations of the rTMS application in SCI patients. First, there is a shortage of studies providing evidences of sustained benefits of rTMS therapy beyond conventional treatments. Besides the different stimulation protocols and parameters applied, type of lesion and nonuniform assessment methodologies hamper the development of consistent evidences. Although evidences so far do not suggest any harm to the subjects, safety issues should be also considered when using rTMS in SCI patients, especially because of the high threshold needed to evoke motor responses in the impaired pathways [16].

More research is needed to provide robust evidence that can support the use of rTMS as an alternative to standard therapies. In addition to bigger sample sizes used in each study, researchers should also test the same (or very similar) stimulation parameters and protocols to provide reproducible results. Finally, it is critical to better understand the pathophysiology of neural structures affected by rTMS to design optimal and customized protocols that might boost beneficial neural changes coupled with functional recovery after SCI [2].

2.2 Transcranial direct current stimulation (tDCS)

Transcranial direct current stimulation (tDCS) is a technology that delivers continuous low current stimulation (1–2 mA) via paired anode and cathode electrodes over the scalp [4, 14, 17] (see **Figure 2**). This modality is usually combined with motor training to promote activity-dependent plasticity [14]. tDCS may change brain function by causing neurons resting potential to depolarize or hyperpolarize. Depolarization happens when positive stimulation (anodal tDCS) is delivered, which increases neural excitability and, therefore, neural firing. Cathodal tDCS (negative stimulation) causes hyperpolarization and, thus, decreases neural firing [4].

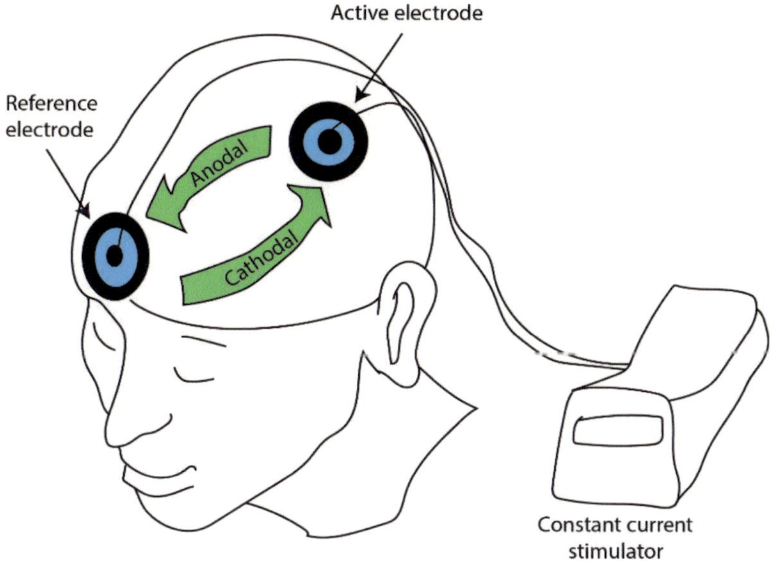

Figure 2.
Transcranial direct current stimulation delivers continuous low current stimulation by applying a positive (anodal) or negative (cathodal) current via paired electrodes over the scalp.

This technique is still in the early stage. To our knowledge, just seven studies have examined improvements in motor function after SCI related to the use of tDCS: four studies evaluated its effect on upper limb function [18–21] and three studies evaluated the tDCS effect on lower limb function and gait [22–24]. All these studies used anodal stimulation and showed improvements in upper and lower limb motor function.

The use of tDCS has led to improvements in pinch force, manual dexterity, and force modulation when combined with repetitive practice [18]. Other study reported that stimulation intensity affects functional outcomes when tDCS was delivered at rest: increased corticospinal excitability to affected muscles was obtained when using 2 mA stimulation, but not 1 mA, in nine chronic SCI patients [19]. Another study also reported gains in hand motor function after a single session of 2mA tDCS, though no improvements were described in clinical scales [20]. When combining tDCS with robot-assisted arm training, SCI patients improved arm and hand function post-treatment and at the 2-month follow-up [21].

The three studies that evaluated the tDCS effect on lower limb function and gait showed improved motor function [22–24]. However, one of these studies combined tDCS with robotic gait training and also showed no significant differences between these improvements and those verified in the group who received sham stimulation combined with robotic gait training [22].

tDCS is an attractive noninvasive modality option for the treatment after SCI: it is affordable and does not present substantial adverse events (when present, they included redness of the skin, sleepiness, headache, and neck pain [4]). However, further research is still needed to provide robust evidence that support the use of tDCS to improve motor function and to be used in the clinical setting as a long-term strategy after SCI.

3. Transcutaneous spinal cord stimulation (tcSCS)

In the recent years, spinal cord electrical stimulation (SCS) has arisen as a promising tool to modulate corticospinal excitability and modify the motor output in

SCI individuals. The most extended form of SCS is epidural SCS, which consists on delivering electrical currents through arrays of electrodes implanted in the epidural space of the spinal cord, in order to modify the excitatory output of the spinal cord. It has been widely studied as an application for chronic pain relief [14]. Promising results from a recent research showed its potential to improve neurological recovery and support the activities of daily living (including walking) after SCI [25].

Transcutaneous spinal cord stimulation (tcSCS) is a novel form of SCS that delivers superficial stimulation, usually over the skin that overlies the lower thoracic and/or lumbosacral vertebrae [26]. The principles underlying tcSCS rely on the physiology of the corticospinal pathways in the spinal cord that can produce excitability changes in the different neural populations of the spinal circuitry [27, 28]. Central pattern generators (CPGs) are pools of neurons able to elicit rhythmic and coordinated movements without the contribution of supraspinal centers. CPGs use proprioceptive information to provide real-time and coordinated control of motor output. The propriospinal system serves as an integratory interface between supraspinal and spinal centers, modulating motor activity. tcSCS is able to modulate the excitability properties of these systems by means of different stimulation protocols, in which the surface array placement along the spinal cord, direction of the current, intensity, frequency, and timing of stimulation result in different modulation outcomes. tcSCS was able to activate GPGs in healthy volunteers, eliciting coordinated and synchronized nonvoluntary movements of the lower limb [28]. These findings have been reproduced in SCI individuals, namely by reactivating damaged spinal circuitries that were previously considered as nonfunctional. When tcSCS was applied over several training sessions in SCI patients, there was improved voluntary modulation of movement of the lower limbs [29]. Moreover, combining tcSCS training with pharmacology therapy and exoskeletons increased motor control enhancement [26].

tcSCS overcomes the invasiveness and costs of epidural SCS with the trade-off of poor spatial stimulation resolution. Although the number of studies using this technique is considerably low, and the exact physiological mechanisms behind the improvements shown are still yet to be fully understood, tcSCS is already a promising tool to be considered in future SCI rehabilitation. Multi-approach therapies including tcSCS, pharmacological, active movement, and robotic-assisted training should be considered to exploit the combination of different physiological effects produced by each modality and maximize motor recovery [26].

4. Peripheral stimulation and assistive devices

Motor control and the execution of voluntary movements require the interaction between afferent feedback and supraspinal input to accurately plan and execute movements. This interplay induces activity-dependent plasticity at both the brain and spinal cord level [30, 31]. After SCI, afferent feedback is impaired and becomes essential to reorganize spinal circuits below the lesion area [30]. Therefore, non-invasive modalities that apply surface electrical stimulation at the peripheral level (either alone or combined with assisted training) to augment or modify neural function are very appealing and have been applied in SCI rehabilitation.

This section overviews two forms of surface stimulation that are user friendly and can be easily administered by a therapist during SCI rehabilitation: transcutaneous electrical nerve stimulation (TENS) and functional electrical stimulation (FES). The second part of this section reports the main results attained when using cycling driven by electrical stimulation and the combination of electrical stimulation with external robotic devices.

4.1 Transcutaneous electrical nerve stimulation (TENS)

TENS is the most common noninvasive modality used in physical therapy [32]. This type of stimulation delivers high-frequency (50–150 Hz) and low-intensity (below motor threshold) surface electrical current [33].

Though TENS has been commonly used in pain control and to reduce muscle stiffness/tone, there are also some reports on decreased spasticity due to the use of this modality. For instance, TENS has recently reduced spasticity in SCI patients and the effects outlasted up to several hours after treatment [34]. This is because TENS activates sensory nerves that in turn may activate inhibitory interneurons that will inhibit the spastic muscle activity [34]. More specifically, these anti-spastic effects are due to the release of gamma-aminobutyric acid (GABA) that acts as inhibitory neurotransmitters, achieving similar anti-spastic effects to those of baclofen [32], which is a first-line treatment for spasticity, especially in adults who suffered a SCI [35]. Results of spasticity treatment using TENS seem to improve when combined with physical therapy [36].

Given its low cost, lack of adverse event effects, and ease to use, TENS seems to be a very good solution to treat spasticity after SCI. Moreover, since TENS alleviates pain and fatigue and can be used for periods of several hours, it seems to be appropriate for the beginning of the rehabilitation after SCI, when training is not very intensive.

4.2 Functional electrical stimulation (FES) and brain-machine interfaces (BMIs)

FES is another modality of electrical stimulation that has become very popular in the clinical setting. FES is similar to TENS in the sense that the two modalities use electrodes on the skin to provide electrical stimulation to a desired location of the body; but they differ in the settings and especially in the purpose of their use. Unlike TENS, FES delivers trains of electrical stimulation above motor threshold to stimulate a muscle or the efferent nerve supplying a muscle in order to attain a muscle contraction [14]. The higher the amplitude of this stimulation, the bigger is the number of recruited efferent fibers and, therefore, the higher the muscle contraction.

FES has been used to restore bladder and bowel control, as well as sexual function, which are ranked among the most important functions to regain among SCI patients [37]. FES has also been widely used for the treatment of muscle weakness, gait training, and muscle reeducation [34]. In the case of SCI, it is well known that artificially induced contraction of weak or paralyzed muscles brings several therapeutic benefits, such as prevention of lower limb muscle atrophy, increased muscle strength, endurance, and cardiovascular fitness [38, 39]. In addition to these benefits, the coordinated stimulation of efferent nerves (usually to stimulate agonist-antagonist muscles of a joint) can be paired with a functional activity to produce a given biomechanical task and, thus, restore motor function [34].

On the other hand, there is evidence that peripheral stimulation, if synchronized with patients' voluntary effort, can further promote recovery [14]. In fact, improved modulation together with volitional control seems to be key factors to reinforce connectivity during rehabilitation of SCI patients, presumably through synaptic enhancement [14]. In this sense, brain-machine interfaces (BMIs) are currently the most sophisticated neuromodulation tools to restore voluntary limb movements after SCI. In the context of the noninvasive modalities described in this chapter, BMIs can be used to stimulate the peripheral nervous system by use of decoded brain signals recorded with electroencephalography (EEG) [14].

Finally, FES has also been used to reduce spasticity in SCI patients, usually by stimulating the spastic muscle. This is hypothesized to modulate recurrent inhibition via Renshaw cells [34]. These inhibitory interneurons are excited by collaterals of the axons of motoneurons and make inhibitory synaptic connections with several populations of motoneurons, including those that excite them [40]. This reciprocal inhibition is important to prevent overshooting muscle contraction induced by FES.

Despite all the benefits here described, FES presents several challenges for tasks that are executed for long periods of time. Limited muscle force generation, rapid onset of muscle fatigue, and nonlinear, time-dependent mechanical responses, as well as the redundancy of the musculoskeletal system are the main challenges of this technology that traditionally hamper generalized use for rehabilitation and/or motor compensation of walking. However, multi-electrode techniques are showing promising results [41] and should be explored.

4.3 FES driven cycling

Physical activity of SCI people whose limbs are paralyzed is very important to maintain their physiological well-being. A promising approach is the application of FES during cycling movements. This technique, called FES cycling, is a noninvasive training protocol used in medical rehabilitation, mostly addressed to individual affected by SCI. This method can be applied continuously for tens of minutes, with direct benefits on muscle strength. Besides muscle strengthening, FES cycling is beneficial for cardiovascular and respiratory functions [42].

FES training for lower limb muscles can be performed on stationary cycle ergometers or mobile tricycles. As shown in **Figure 3**, FES is managed by a controller, which receives signals from a crank angle sensor and, depending on the actual crank position, transfers sequences of electrical impulses to surface electrodes to stimulate muscles and generate active muscle force. The power output produced by the application of FES depends on three main aspects. The first is the number of muscle groups stimulated. The second is the parameters of the stimulating current, that is, amplitude, pulse width, and frequency. The third is the timing of the stimulating signal sent to the individual muscles.

FES cycling is usually applied on several lower limb muscles simultaneously [43]. The main muscle groups considered are the hamstrings and quadriceps and, in

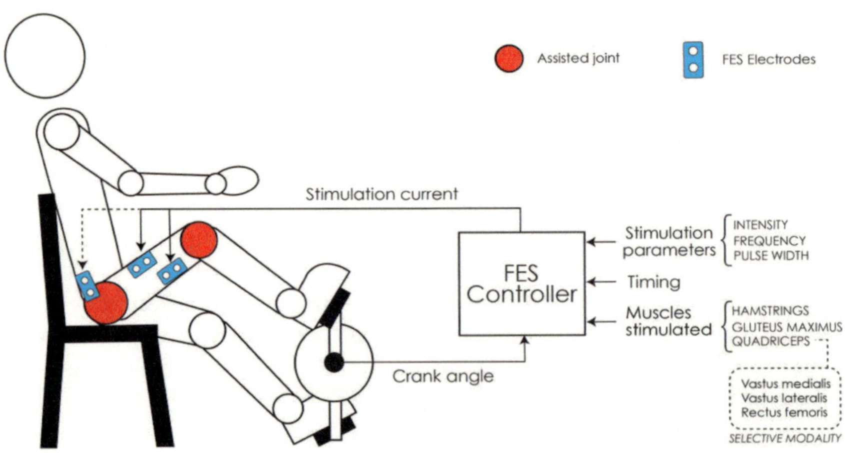

Figure 3.
FES driven cycling: a controller sends electrical signals (stimulation current) to selected muscles. The actual muscle forces depend on the actual crank angle value transferred to the controller and on the parameters and timing of the stimulation signals sent to individual muscles.

some cases, the gluteus maximus. The quadriceps are stimulated either as a whole, that is, using only one pair of electrodes, or more selectively, in which three muscles composing them—that is, the vastus medialis, vastus lateralis, and rectus femoris—are stimulated individually. This more selective stimulation has demonstrated, in a recent pilot study, to improve up to 27% the power output in one patient with spastic muscles [44]. In this case, while the total stimulation current (the sum of the amplitude of currents applied in all of the channels) was higher, lower stimulation current amplitudes per muscle groups were sufficient to generate the required movement. The average current amplitude applied in FES cycling in SCI individuals is around 50–70 mA per muscles and it varies in a wide range. In some protocols, the current amplitude is increased until 120–140 mA to achieve power output around 10 W [45] and in extreme cases 20 W [46]. Others stimulated muscles with a frequency of 30 Hz, current amplitude of 70–90 mA, and pulse width of 500 μs, reaching a power output around 30 W [47]. The timing of stimulation is usually set according to recorded and processed muscle activities of able-bodied persons and/or on physiological, biomechanical parameters of the muscles and limbs of the participants. Nevertheless, these approaches are either not adaptive to the patient-specific musculoskeletal conditions, or very difficult to calibrate. For instance, when applying selective stimulation of the three quadriceps muscles separately [44], we found that the participant, even reaching higher power output, preferred to cycle for a shorter time, possibly due to a nonphysiological stimulation strategy. In our opinion, more studies are needed to explore these control combinations, in particular considering the case of selective stimulation. This will likely lead to new more efficient, natural, and adaptable stimulation protocols.

Cadence is another important variable in FES-cycling rehabilitation. In the case of ergometer-based training, cadence is on average set to 45–50 rpm, in most of the stimulating conditions. To adapt the treatment to patient residual motor ability, cadence can be changed in combination with various crank resistances during the rehabilitation process. Tricycles have been proposed as an alternative to stationary cycle ergometers [48]. A recent study reported that the series of FES trainings on a tricycle resulted in increased speed of cycling of paraplegics with denervated muscles [49], which is normally not observed in similar ergometer-based protocols. FES-driven tricycling is gaining relevance, as testified by several competitions organized during the last couple of years [50–53]. However, these competitions are only targeting people with SCI. We expect that wider range of participants, for example, stroke, will also be addressed in the near future, as supported by recent promising research works in this direction [54, 55].

4.4 Exoskeletons and hybrid exoskeletons

Repetitive and intensive task-specific training drives beneficial neuroplasticity, thus enhancing functional recovery [56]. Therefore, exoskeletons for motor rehabilitation purposes have emerged in the last decade as a convenient technology that allow multiple, intensive, and more effective sessions of gait training, allowing SCI patients to ameliorate their performance in daily life [56]. Moreover, a study reported that spasticity and pain intensity of SCI patients decreased after one single session of walking assisted by a powered robotic exoskeleton [56].

A paradigmatic development of a stationary rehabilitation robot for gait training is the Lokomat system, which combines body-weight supported treadmill-training (BWSTT) with the assistance of a robotic gait orthosis. These robotic systems are able to provide guidance forces to the lower limb segments to induce a consisting stepping pattern with adjustable guidance. It has been shown that although the mechanical coupling and added guidance may change the task constraints and in turn alter voluntary leg movements, the basic neuromuscular pattern is preserved when intact humans walk assisted by this robot [57]. Robot-assisted gait training with the Lokomat after SCI has been shown in some studies to improve outcomes related to mobility when compared to conventional overground training [58, 59]. For example, it was shown improved gait distance, strength, and functional level of mobility and independence of acute SCI patients receiving robotic-assisted gait training than the group of patients receiving conventional overground training [60]. Also, it has been demonstrated that robot-assisted gait training combined with conventional physiotherapy could yield more improvement in ambulatory function of SCI patients than conventional therapy alone. However, the impact of such complementary tools to provide neuromuscular education is still not well established for a convincing penetration of these systems in the clinical rehabilitation environments. Some limitations of such stationary robotic tools are that robotic-assisted training can be limited in the range of gait speed at which the exoskeleton robot can provide a comfortable gait pattern. Also, the stationary machine imposes restrictions to the user movements to the sagittal plane, significantly preventing motion in the frontal and transversal plane that are required for overground walking.

Wearable robots (WR) for overground untethered assisted walking are emerging devices that have the potential to overcome some of the above-mentioned constraints and opening a range of clinical application scenarios. Through wearable mechanical actuation and sensing, WRs are proliferating for their use as assistive and rehabilitation technologies due to their ability to replicate the complex motions involved in human movement. As a result, the past few decades have seen an increasing amount of research focused on developing robotic systems intended to interact with the neurologically impaired human body. This interaction (of the human body) with WRs has been established in foundational literature [61] as dual, bidirectional physical (pHRi), and cognitive (cHRi) interactions. While these systems have been proven to be useful for specific applications, such as in-clinic rehabilitation, current research in the area of pHRi for WRs is focusing more on developing lightweight and flexible force interactions with hardware solutions that might be more suitable to a broader range of applications (by adding compliance to rigid exoskeletons [62, 63] or developing "soft exosuits" [64]). However, these soft exoskeletons are in early stage and the majority of clinical evidence of their efficacy for treatment of SCI is in studies with motorized powered exoskeletons. A systematic review of the literature on powered WRs for overground gait rehabilitation pointed out that, although current technology is still under development, and hence its ultimate impact remains still unclear, a number of revised studies report positive changes in outcome variables and suggest that training time and improvements in gait speed using powered WRs are correlated in SCI population [65].

On the cHRi side, efforts are focused on developing means for interpretation of mechanical and neural signals to establish adequate control methods that integrate WRs as parts of human functioning. In this regard, a scheme for "symbiotic interaction" between humans and WRs has been recently developed in the FET Project BioMot (FP7-ICT-2013-10-611695), yielding new technologies to interface human neuromechanics with robot-control algorithms to guide assistance; the point of increasing their proficiency is to make them more capable of sophisticated interdependent joint activity with the human wearer. Under this approach, a tacit adaptability is provided to modulate the compliance in the robot torque controller, to automatically modulate in turn the difficulty of the task [66].

There is currently no agreement on the optimal robot-mediated treatment programs to induce plasticity and promote recovery of motor function following SCI, and the understanding of recovery mechanisms is still an open matter [67]. Whatever the robot hardware and patient's functional status, a WR-mediated neurorehabilitation model could pave the way for effective restoration of mobility after major neurological conditions. In the last few years, the development of computational neurorehabilitation models is becoming a relevant topic in the domain of neural repair, as these computational models can be expected to provide the basis for future clinical robot software that suggests timing, dosage, and content of therapy. For example, an analytical modeling approach has been applied to robot-mediated rehabilitation data of a group of SCI subjects, providing insights with regard to patient grouping and gait recovery prognosis and also providing predictive quantitative measures to consider before starting the treatment [68]. This, together with the fact that in the past years we are witnessing an unprecedented number of wearable interactive robotics products that will populate even more the clinic environments, a reasonable long-term vision is to gather multicenter clinical data to equip rehabilitation WRs with computational neurorehabilitation modeling tools that will in turn provide enriched data to establish scientific bases of exoskeleton-guided recovery.

On the other hand, the combination of FES with external orthotic devices that provide joint support and mechanical constraint to undesired movements was early proposed [69], but the challenges associated with the rapid onset of muscle fatigue and movement control still remained. In an attempt to further diminish the energy demand from the muscle while providing better joint control, FES systems were combined with lower limb exoskeletons, also called hybrid exoskeletons [70]. The combination of the lower limb robotic exoskeleton and the FES system can be shaped in different ways, depending on the configuration of the FES system and/or the exoskeleton. Regarding the former, the FES can be implanted [71] or superficial [72] and can be found either under open [71, 73] or closed-loop [72, 74] control of stimulation. With regards to the exoskeleton joints, it can provide means of dissipating energy, via the use of clutches or brakes [75, 76], or can feature active joints, which can also provide energy to the joints.

The hybrid configuration presents some advantages with respect to the FES or exoskeleton applications alone. First, the exoskeleton structure provides passive control to the joints, constraining undesirable movements. The actuators can provide support to the joints, diminishing or eliminating the need for stimulation of certain muscles (e.g., quadriceps muscles during the stance phases of walking). In the case of active actuators, the movement produced by the FES is supported by the actuator, improving the control of the joint trajectory while delaying muscle fatigue [77]. On the other hand, the sensors of the exoskeleton provide information for closing the control loop of the FES system, which may further help on optimizing the performance of the muscle in terms of either force production or muscle fatigue [72].

Despite hybrid exoskeletons show several advantages, the field is not mature. There is a markedly low activity in this field, and most of the groups working on this technology have discontinued their research on this topic. The rationale for this may come from the bottlenecks of each technology. First, hybrid exoskeletons share drawbacks with lower limb robotic exoskeletons, in which the combination with a FES system add complexity on the control and wearing aspects. Besides, although alleviated by the exoskeleton, the nonlinear muscle response of the stimulated muscles and the muscle fatigue is not adequately solved yet, and eventually all hybrid exoskeletons still have to be designed to function as conventional robotic exoskeletons once muscle fatigue appears.

Lastly, there is a need of conducting clinical studies that can demonstrate the benefits of using hybrid exoskeleton with respect to exoskeleton alone that actually justify the extra complexity, cost, and cumbersomeness of the FES system.

5. Conclusions and future directions

This chapter presents an overview of the main effects on motor and functional recovery, as well as spasticity and pain, when using a wide range of noninvasive modalities in the rehabilitation of SCI patients, either in the research or the clinical setting. According to the level of stimulation, these modalities were divided into three different sections: brain, spinal cord, and peripheral stimulation. Regarding the last one, stimulation of the peripheral nervous system can also be combined with external devices that assist and allow repetitive motor training (e.g., hybrid exoskeletons and FES driven cycling).

Noninvasive brain stimulation (NIBS) techniques such as rTMS and tDCS have the potential to improve motor function recovery and spasticity after SCI. Moreover, NIBS techniques are safe and relatively easy to administer, presenting infrequent mild effects. Very few studies have investigated motor function after delivery of rTMS on SCI patients. Improvements seem to be present when higher rTMS frequencies are used. On the other hand, the few studies that investigated the effects of rTMS on spasticity in iSCI reported some reduction in the clinical symptoms of spasticity [2]. There are less studies of the application of tDCS in motor function or spasticity than those of rTMS [4], though they all showed improvements in upper or lower limb motor function. Thus, more research is needed to address the full potential and incorporate NIBS techniques into SCI rehabilitation [4].

At the spinal level stimulation, tcSCS has irrupted in the last years as a neurorehabilitation tool in SCI. It overcomes the limitation of invasiveness and costs of epidural stimulation at the expense of poor spatial stimulation resolution. The few evidences suggest that tsSCS alone improves voluntary modulation of lower limb movement [29] and increases motor control enhancement when combined with pharmacology therapy and exoskeletons [26].

Noninvasive modalities that deliver different types of surface stimulation at the peripheral level (either alone or combined with cycling or robotic-assisted training, for example) are very appealing and have been applied in SCI rehabilitation. Surface electrical stimulation can modulate afferent and efferent pathways in order to induce corticospinal plasticity. For instance, TENS and FES have reduced spasticity in SCI patients and the effects outlasted up to several hours after treatment, though the two techniques target different nerve groups in order to reduce spasticity: TENS activates afferents that in turn activate inhibitory interneurons that will inhibit the spastic muscle activity; FES induces muscle contraction and is oriented to the spastic muscle [34]. The development of fatigue and discomfort produced by the intensity of stimulation of FES is a drawback for long sessions. Thus, TENS may be appropriate for the beginning of the rehabilitation, while FES may have better effects on those SCI patients presenting spasmodic behavior [34]. On the other hand, BMIs may enhance brain and spinal cord neurorecovery through activity dependent plasticity. Future advances in wireless devices may potentiate the widespread use of BMIs in the clinical setting.

FES cycling is another modality that presents direct benefits on muscle strength, as well as cardiovascular and respiratory functions of SCI patients. However, more research on this technique is needed in order to design more efficient, natural, and adaptable stimulation protocols, which will likely improve motor function outcomes during SCI rehabilitation.

Robotic devices, such as exoskeletons, are other solutions that have been used for rehabilitation purposed after SCI. These devices can provide intensive, long lasting repetitive task specific training to SCI patients, which is the principle behind motor rehabilitation and beneficial neuroplasticity [78]. These devices have allowed SCI patients to ameliorate their performance in daily life [56]. The hybrid configuration (exoskeleton combined with FES) presents some advantages with respect to the FES or exoskeleton applications alone: actuators can provide support to the joints, diminishing or eliminating the need for stimulation of certain muscles; the sensors of the exoskeleton provide information for closing the control loop of the FES system, which may further help on optimizing the performance of the muscle in terms of either force production or muscle fatigue. However, the field is not mature and there is a need of conducting clinical studies that can demonstrate the benefits of using hybrid exoskeleton with respect to exoskeleton alone that actually justify the extra complexity, cost, and cumbersomeness of the FES system.

Part of the current SCI rehabilitation research uses the modalities described in this chapter and has presented promising results including neurorecovery.

Some of these modalities are already being widely introduced into the clinical rehabilitation of SCI, such as TENS and FES. However, the actual uptake of technology in the clinical setting, especially for SCI rehabilitation, has been very low [5]. There are still some barriers to the clinical implementation of these techniques. Three of those barriers are the feasibility, appropriateness, and the cost. While the research here described is practical for SCI rehabilitation, some of these techniques are less practicable: they require specialized equipment and knowledge, which make them less feasible [5]. Despite the scientific evidence in favor of these technologies, the expertise required to operate and repair emerging technology is usually not found in the clinical setting, which makes it less appropriate. A third barrier that deserves attention is the economic cost, given the fact that most of the clinical centers cannot afford the maintenance of these technologies. To overcome these barriers, it is essential to develop a proactive dialog between researchers and clinicians in order to properly examine each of the emerging modalities that can maximize the outcomes for each individual that suffered a SCI.

Acknowledgements

This work was funded by the European Union's Horizon 2020 research and innovation programme (Project EXTEND—Bidirectional Hyper-Connected Neural System) under grant agreement No 779982 and by the EFOP-3.6.1-16-2016-00004 grant.

Conflict of interest

The authors declare that this work was conducted in the absence of any commercial or financial relationships that could be considered as a potential conflict of interest.

Author details

Filipe O. Barroso[1*], Alejandro Pascual-Valdunciel[1], Diego Torricelli[1], Juan C. Moreno[1], Antonio Del Ama-Espinosa[2], Jozsef Laczko[3,4] and José L. Pons[1]

1 Neural Rehabilitation Group, Cajal Institute, Spanish National Research Council (CSIC), Madrid, Spain

2 Biomechanics and Assistive Technology Unit, National Hospital for Paraplegics, Toledo, Spain

3 Department of Information Technology and Biorobotics, Faculty of Science, University of Pecs, Hungary

4 Hungarian Academy of Sciences, Wigner Research Centre for Physics, Hungary

*Address all correspondence to: filipe.barroso@cajal.csic.es

References

[1] Barroso FO, Torricelli D, Bravo-Esteban E, Taylor J, Gómez-Soriano J, Santos C, et al. Muscle synergies in cycling after incomplete spinal cord injury: Correlation with clinical measures of motor function and spasticity. Frontiers in Human Neuroscience. 2016;**9**(706). DOI: 10.3389/fnhum.2015.00706

[2] Tazoe T, Perez MA. Effects of repetitive transcranial magnetic stimulation on recovery of function after spinal cord injury. Archives of Physical Medicine and Rehabilitation. 2015;**96**(4 Suppl):S145-S155. DOI: 10.1016/j.apmr.2014.07.418

[3] van Middendorp JJ, Allison HC, Ahuja S, Bracher D, Dyson C, Fairbank J, et al. Top ten research priorities for spinal cord injury: The methodology and results of a British priority setting partnership. Spinal Cord. 2016;**54**(5):341-346. DOI: 10.1038/sc.2015.199

[4] Gunduz A, Rothwell J, Vidal J, Kumru H. Non-invasive brain stimulation to promote motor and functional recovery following spinal cord injury. Neural Regeneration Research. 2017;**12**(12):1933-1938. DOI: 10.4103/1673-5374.221143

[5] Musselman KE, Shah M, Zariffa J. Rehabilitation technologies and interventions for individuals with spinal cord injury: Translational potential of current trends. Journal of Neuroengineering and Rehabilitation. 2018;**15**(40). DOI: 10.1186/s12984-018-0386-7

[6] Ganguly K, Poo MM. Activity-dependent neural plasticity from bench to bedside. Neuron. 2013;**80**(3):729-741. DOI: 10.1016/j.neuron.2013.10.028

[7] Ramón y Cajal S. Estudios sobre la degeneración y regeneración del Sistema nervioso. Madrid: Imprenta de Hijos de Nicolás Moya; 1913

[8] Hebb DO. The Organization of Behavior: A Neuropsychological Theory. New York: Wiley; 1949

[9] Tahayori B, Koceja DM. Activity-dependent plasticity of spinal circuits in the developing and mature spinal cord. Neural Plasticity. 2012;**2012**. DOI: 10.1155/2012/964843

[10] Onifer SM, Smith GM, Fouad K. Plasticity after spinal cord injury: Relevance to recovery and approaches to facilitate it. Neurotherapeutics. 2011;**8**(2):283-293. DOI: 10.1007/s13311-011-0034-4

[11] Mawase F, Uehara S, Bastian AJ, Celnik P. Motor learning enhances use-dependent plasticity. The Journal of Neuroscience. 2017;**37**(10):2673-2685. DOI: 10.1523/JNEUROSCI.3303-16.2017

[12] Barroso FO, Torricelli D, Moreno JC. Emerging techniques for assessment of sensorimotor impairments after spinal cord injury. In: Fuller H, Gates M, editors. Recovery of Motor Function Following Spinal Cord Injury. London: IntechOpen; 2016. pp. 305-322. DOI: 10.5772/64182

[13] Squair JW, Bjerkefors A, Inglis JT, Lam T, Carpenter MG. Cortical and vestibular stimulation reveal preserved descending motor pathways in individuals with motor-complete spinal cord injury. Journal of Rehabilitation Medicine. 2016;**48**(7):589-596. DOI: 10.2340/16501977-2101

[14] James ND, McMahon SB, Field-Fote EC, Bradbury EJ. Neuromodulation in the restoration of function after spinal cord injury. Lancet Neurology. 2018;**17**(10):905-917. DOI: 10.1016/S1474-4422(18)30287-4

[15] Rossini PM, Burke D, Chen R, Cohen LG, Daskalakis Z, Di Iorio R, et al. Non-invasive electrical and magnetic stimulation of the brain, spinal cord, roots and peripheral nerves: Basic principles and procedures for routine clinical and research application. An updated report from an I.F.C.N. Committee. Clinical Neurophysiology. 2015;**126**(6):1071-1107. DOI: 10.1016/j.clinph.2015.02.001

[16] Ellaway PH, Vásquez N, Craggs M. Induction of central nervous system plasticity by repetitive transcranial magnetic stimulation to promote sensorimotor recovery in incomplete spinal cord injury. Frontiers in Integrative Neuroscience. 2014;**8**(42). DOI: 10.3389/fnint.2014.00042

[17] Nitsche MA, Liebetanz D, Lang N, Antal A, Tergau F, Paulus W. Safety criteria for transcranial direct current stimulation (tDCS) in humans. Clinical Neurophysiology. 2003;**114**(11):2220-2222

[18] Gomes-Osman J, Field-Fote EC. Cortical vs. afferent stimulation as an adjunct to functional task practice training: A randomized, comparative pilot study in people with cervical spinal cord injury. Clinical Rehabilitation. 2015;**29**(8):771-782. DOI: 10.1177/0269215514556087

[19] Murray LM, Edwards DJ, Ruffini G, Labar D, Stampas A, Pascual-Leone A, et al. Intensity dependent effects of transcranial direct current stimulation on corticospinal excitability in chronic spinal cord injury. Archives of Physical Medicine and Rehabilitation. 2015;**96** (4 Suppl):S114-S121. DOI: 10.1016/j.apmr.2014.11.004

[20] Cortes M, Medeiros AH, Gandhi A, Lee P, Krebs HI, Thickbroom G, et al. Improved grasp function with transcranial direct current stimulation in chronic spinal cord injury. NeuroRehabilitation. 2017;**41**(1):51-59. DOI: 10.3233/NRE-171456

[21] Yozbatiran N, Keser Z, Davis M, Stampas A, O'Malley MK, Cooper-Hay C, et al. Transcranial direct current stimulation (tDCS) of the primary motor cortex and robot-assisted arm training in chronic incomplete cervical spinal cord injury: A proof of concept sham-randomized clinical study. NeuroRehabilitation. 2016;**39**(3): 401-411. DOI: 10.3233/NRE-161371

[22] Kumru H, Murillo N, Benito-Penalva J, Tormos JM, Vidal J. Transcranial direct current stimulation is not effective in the motor strength and gait recovery following motor incomplete spinal cord injury during Lokomat(®) gait training. Neuroscience Letters. 2016;**620**:143-147. DOI: 10.1016/j.neulet.2016.03.056

[23] Raithatha R, Carrico C, Powell ES, Westgate PM, Chelette Ii KC, Lee K, et al. Non-invasive brain stimulation and robot-assisted gait training after incomplete spinal cord injury: A randomized pilot study. NeuroRehabilitation. 2016;**38**(1):15-25. DOI: 10.3233/NRE-151291

[24] Yamaguchi T, Fujiwara T, Tsai YA, Tang SC, Kawakami M, Mizuno K, et al. The effects of anodal transcranial direct current stimulation and patterned electrical stimulation on spinal inhibitory interneurons and motor function in patients with spinal cord injury. Experimental Brain Research. 2016;**234**(6):1469-1478. DOI: 10.1007/s00221-016-4561-4

[25] Wagner FB, Mignardot JB, Le Goff-Mignardot CG, Demesmaeker R, Komi S, Capogrosso M, et al. Targeted neurotechnology restores walking in humans with spinal cord injury. Nature. 2018;**563**(7729):65-71. DOI: 10.1038/s41586-018-0649-2

[26] Gerasimenko Y, Gorodnichev R, Moshonkina T, Sayenko D, Gad P, Reggie Edgerton V. Transcutaneous electrical spinal-cord stimulation in humans. Annals of Physical

and Rehabilitation Medicine. 2015;**58**(4):225-231. DOI: 10.1016/j.rehab.2015.05.003

[27] Nardone R, Höller Y, Taylor A, Thomschewski A, Oriol A, Frey V, et al. Noninvasive spinal cord stimulation: Technical aspects and therapeutic applications. Neuromodulation. 2015;**18**(7):580-591. DOI: 10.1111/ner.12332

[28] Taccola G, Sayenko D, Gad P, Gerasimenko Y, Edgerton VR. And yet it moves: Recovery of volitional control after spinal cord injury. Progress in Neurobiology. 2018;**160**:64-81. DOI: 10.1016/j.pneurobio.2017.10.004

[29] Gerasimenko YP, Lu DC, Modaber M, Zdunowski S, Gad P, Sayenko DG, et al. Noninvasive reactivation of motor descending control after paralysis. Journal of Neurotrauma. 2015;**32**(24):1968-1980. DOI: 10.1089/neu.2015.4008

[30] Piazza S, Serrano-Muñoz D, Gómez-Soriano J, Torricelli D, Segura-Fragosa A, Pons JL, et al. Afferent electrical stimulation during cycling improves spinal processing of sensorimotor function after incomplete spinal cord injury. NeuroRehabilitation. 2017;**40**(3):429-437. DOI: 10.3233/NRE-161430

[31] Wolpaw JR. Spinal cord plasticity in acquisition and maintenance of motor skills. Acta Physiologica (Oxford, England). 2007;**189**(2):155-169. DOI: 10.1111/j.1748-1716.2006.01656.x

[32] Manigandan G, Bharathi K. Effect of transcutaneous electrical nerve stimulation over gastrocnemius muscle spasticity among hemiparetic patients. Journal of Physiotherapy Research. 2017;**1**(2)

[33] Fernández-Tenorio E, Serrano-Muñoz D, Avendaño-Coy J, Gómez-Soriano J. Transcutaneous electrical nerve stimulation for spasticity: A systematic review. Neurología. 2016. DOI: 10.1016/j.nrl.2016.06.009

[34] Sivaramakrishnan A, Solomon JM, Manikandan N. Comparison of transcutaneous electrical nerve stimulation (TENS) and functional electrical stimulation (FES) for spasticity in spinal cord injury—A pilot randomized cross-over trial. The Journal of Spinal Cord Medicine. 2018;**41**(4):397-406. DOI: 10.1080/10790268.2017.1390930

[35] Chang E, Ghosh N, Yanni D, Lee S, Alexandru D, Mozaffar T. A review of spasticity treatments: Pharmacological and interventional approaches. Critical Reviews in Physical and Rehabilitation Medicine. 2013;**25**(1-2):11-22. DOI: 10.1615/CritRevPhysRehabilMed.2013007945

[36] Mills PB, Dossa F. Transcutaneous electrical nerve stimulation for management of limb spasticity: A systematic review. American Journal of Physical Medicine & Rehabilitation. 2016;**95**(4):309-318. DOI: 10.1097/PHM.0000000000000437

[37] Creasey GH, Craggs MD. Functional electrical stimulation for bladder, bowel, and sexual function. Handbook of Clinical Neurology. 2012;**109**:247-257. DOI: 10.1016/B978-0-444-52137-8.00015-2

[38] Thrasher TA, Popovic MR. Functional electrical stimulation of walking: Function, exercise and rehabilitation. Annales de Réadaptation et de Médecine Physique. 2008;**51**(6):452-460. DOI: 10.1016/j.annrmp.2008.05.006

[39] Nightingale EJ, Raymond J, Middleton JW, Crosbie J, Davis GM. Benefits of FES gait in a spinal cord injured population. Spinal Cord. 2007;**45**(10):646-657. DOI: 10.1038/sj.sc.3102101

[40] Kandel ER, Schwartz JH, Jessell TM, Siegelbaum SA, Hudspeth AJ. Principles

of Neural Science. 5h ed. McGraw-Hill Education/Medical; 2013

[41] Koutsou AD, Moreno JC, Del Ama AJ, Rocon E, Pons JL. Advances in selective activation of muscles for non-invasive motor neuroprostheses. Journal of Neuroengineering and Rehabilitation. 2016;**13**(56). DOI: 10.1186/s12984-016-0165-2

[42] Hunt KJ, Ferrario C, Grant S, Stone B, McLean AN, Fraser MH, et al. Comparison of stimulation patterns for FES-cycling using measures of oxygen cost and stimulation cost. Medical Engineering & Physics. 2006;**28**(7):710-718. DOI: 10.1016/j.medengphy.2005.10.006

[43] Laczko J, Mravcsik M, Katona P. Control of cycling limb movements: Aspects for rehabilitation. Advances in Experimental Medicine and Biology. 2016;**957**:273-289. DOI: 10.1007/978-3-319-47313-0_15

[44] Mravcsik M, Klauber A, Laczko J. FES driven lower limb cycling by four and eight channel stimulations—A comparison in a case study. In: 12th Vienna International Workshop on Functional Electrical Stimulation. Proceedings Book. 2016. pp. 89-93

[45] Theisen D, Fornusek C, Raymond J, Davis GM. External power output changes during prolonged cycling with electrical stimulation. Journal of Rehabilitation Medicine. 2002;**34**(4):171-175

[46] Eser PC, Donaldson Nde N, Knecht H, Stüssi E. Influence of different stimulation frequencies on power output and fatigue during FES-cycling in recently injured SCI people. IEEE Transactions on Neural Systems and Rehabilitation Engineering. 2003;**11**(3):236-240. DOI: 10.1109/TNSRE.2003.817677

[47] Szecsi J, Straube A, Fornusek C. A biomechanical cause of low power production during FES cycling of subjects with SCI. Journal of Neuroengineering and Rehabilitation. 2014;**11**:123. DOI: 10.1186/1743-0003-11-123

[48] Mayr W, Hofer C, Bijak M, Rafolt D, Unger E, Reichel M, et al. Functional electrical stimulation (FES) of denervated muscles: Existing and prospective technological solutions. Basic and Applied Myology. 2002;**12**(6):287-290

[49] Mravcsik M, Kast C, Vargas Luna JL, Aramphianlert W, Hofer C, Malik SZ, et al. FES driven cycling by denervated muscles. In: 22th Annual Conference of the Functional Electrical Stimulation Society. 2018. pp. 134-136

[50] Azevedo Coste C, Wolf P. FES-cycling at cybathlon 2016: Overview on teams and results. Artificial Organs. 2018;**42**(3):336-341. DOI: 10.1111/aor.13139

[51] Berkelmans R, Woods B. Strategies and performances of functional electrical stimulation cycling using the BerkelBike with spinal cord injury in a competition context (CYBATHLON). European Journal of Translational Myology. 2017;**27**(4):255-258. DOI: 10.4081/ejtm.2017.7189

[52] Metani A, Popović-Maneski L, Mateo S, Lemahieu L, Bergeron V. Functional electrical stimulation cycling strategies tested during preparation for the First Cybathlon Competition—A practical report from team ENS de Lyon. European Journal of Translational Myology. 2017;**27**(4):279-288. DOI: 10.4081/ejtm.2017.7110

[53] Fattal C, Sijobert B, Daubigney A, Fachin-Martins E, Lucas B, Casillas JM, et al. Training with FES-assisted cycling in a subject with spinal cord injury: Psychological, physical and physiological considerations. The Journal of Spinal Cord

Medicine. 2018:1-12. DOI: 10.1080/10790268.2018.1490098

[54] Peri E, Ambrosini E, Pedrocchi A, Ferrigno G, Nava C, Longoni V, et al. Can FES-augmented active cycling training improve locomotion in post-acute elderly stroke patients? European Journal of Translational Myology. 2016;**26**(3):187-192. DOI: 10.4081/ejtm.2016.6063

[55] Wang X, Leung KW, Fang Y, Chen S, Tong RK. Design of functional electrical stimulation cycling system for lower-limb rehabilitation of stroke patients. Conference Proceedings—IEEE Engineering in Medicine and Biology Society. 2018:2337-2340. DOI: 10.1109/EMBC.2018.8512869

[56] Stampacchia G, Rustici A, Bigazzi S, Gerini A, Tombini T, Mazzoleni S. Walking with a powered robotic exoskeleton: Subjective experience, spasticity and pain in spinal cord injured persons. NeuroRehabilitation. 2016;**39**(2):277-283. DOI: 10.3233/NRE-161358

[57] Moreno JC, Barroso FO, Farina D, Gizzi L, Santos C, Molinari M, et al. Effects of robotic guidance on the coordination of locomotion. Journal of Neuroengineering and Rehabilitation. 2013;**10**:79. DOI: 10.1186/1743-0003-10-79

[58] Hornby TG, Zemon DH, Campbell D. Robotic-assisted, body-weight-supported treadmill training in individuals following motor incomplete spinal cord injury. Physical Therapy. 2005;**85**(1):52-66

[59] Esclarín-Ruz A, Alcobendas-Maestro M, Casado-Lopez R, Perez-Mateos G, Florido-Sanchez MA, Gonzalez-Valdizan E, et al. A comparison of robotic walking therapy and conventional walking therapy in individuals with upper versus lower motor neuron lesions: A randomized controlled trial. Archives of Physical Medicine and Rehabilitation. 2014;**95**(6):1023-1031. DOI: 10.1016/j.apmr.2013.12.017

[60] Nam KY, Kim HJ, Kwon BS, Park JW, Lee HJ, Yoo A. Robot-assisted gait training (Lokomat) improves walking function and activity in people with spinal cord injury: A systematic review. Journal of Neuroengineering and Rehabilitation. 2017;**14**(1). DOI: 10.1186/s12984-017-0232-3

[61] Pons JL. Wearable Robots: Biomechatronic Exoskeletons. John Wiley & Sons; 2008

[62] Karavas NC, Tsagarakis NG, Saglia J, Galdwell DG. A novel actuator with reconfigurable stiffness for a knee exoskeleton: Design and modeling. In: Advances in Reconfigurable Mechanisms and Robots I. Springer; 2012. pp. 411-421. DOI: 10.1007/978-1-4471-4141-9_37

[63] Bortole M, Venkatakrishnan A, Zhu F, Moreno JC, Francisco GE, Pons JL, et al. The H2 robotic exoskeleton for gait rehabilitation after stroke: Early findings from a clinical study. Journal of Neuroengineering and Rehabilitation. 2015;**12**(54). DOI: 10.1186/s12984-015-0048-y

[64] Polygerinos P, Galloway KC, Savage E, Herman M, O'Donnell K, Walsh CJ. Soft robotic glove for hand rehabilitation and task specific training. In: 2015 IEEE International Conference on Robotics and Automation (ICRA). 2015. pp. 2913-2919. DOI: 10.1109/ICRA.2015.7139597

[65] Contreras-Vidal JL, Bhagat NA, Brantley J, Cruz-Garza JG, He Y, Manley Q, et al. Powered exoskeletons for bipedal locomotion after spinal cord injury. Journal of Neural Engineering. 2016;**13**(3). DOI: 10.1088/1741-2560/13/3/031001

[66] Asín-Prieto G, Martínez-Expósito A, Alnajjar F, Shimoda S, Pons JL, Moreno JC. Feasibility of submaximal force control training for robot–mediated therapy after stroke. In: Converging Clinical and Engineering Research on Neurorehabilitation III; 2019. pp. 256-260. DOI: 10.1007/978-3-030-01845-0_51

[67] Gassert R, Dietz V. Rehabilitation robots for the treatment of sensorimotor deficits: A neurophysiological perspective. Journal of Neuroengineering and Rehabilitation. 2018;**15**(1). DOI: 10.1186/s12984-018-0383-x

[68] Niu X, Varoqui D, Kindig M, Mirbagheri MM. Prediction of gait recovery in spinal cord injured individuals trained with robotic gait orthosis. Journal of Neuroengineering and Rehabilitation. 2014;**11**:42. DOI: 10.1186/1743-0003-11-42

[69] Andrews BJ, Baxendale RH, Barnett R, Phillips GF, Yamazaki T, Paul JP, et al. Hybrid FES orthosis incorporating closed loop control and sensory feedback. Journal of Biomedical Engineering. 1988;**10**(2):189-195

[70] del-Ama AJ, Koutsou AD, Moreno JC, de-los-Reyes A, Gil-Agudo A, Pons JL. Review of hybrid exoskeletons to restore gait following spinal cord injury. Journal of Rehabilitation Research and Development. 2012;**49**(4):497-514

[71] Kobetic R, Marsolais EB, Triolo RJ, Davy DT, Gaudio R, Tashman S. Development of a hybrid gait orthosis: A case report. The Journal of Spinal Cord Medicine. 2003;**26**(3):254-258

[72] del-Ama AJ, Gil-Agudo A, Pons JL, Moreno JC. Hybrid FES-robot cooperative control of ambulatory gait rehabilitation exoskeleton. Journal of Neuroengineering and Rehabilitation. 2014;**11**:27. DOI: 10.1186/1743-0003-11-27

[73] Ha KH, Murray SA, Goldfarb M. An approach for the cooperative control of FES with a powered exoskeleton during level walking for persons with paraplegia. IEEE Transactions on Neural Systems and Rehabilitation Engineering. 2016;**24**(4):455-466. DOI: 10.1109/TNSRE.2015.2421052

[74] Kurokawa N, Yamamoto N, Tagawa Y, Yamamoto T, Kuno H. Development of hybrid FES walking assistive system—Feasibility study. In: The 2012 International Conference on Advanced Mechatronic Systems. 2012. pp. 93-97

[75] Goldfarb M, Durfee WK. Design of a controlled-brake orthosis for FES-aided gait. IEEE Transactions on Rehabilitation Engineering. 1996;**4**(1):13-24

[76] Gharooni S, Heller B, Tokhi MO. A new hybrid spring brake orthosis for controlling hip and knee flexion in the swing phase. IEEE Transactions on Neural Systems and Rehabilitation Engineering. 2001;**9**(1):106-107

[77] Goldfarb M, Korkowski K, Harrold B, Durfee W. Preliminary evaluation of a controlled-brake orthosis for FES-aided gait. IEEE Transactions on Neural Systems and Rehabilitation Engineering. 2003;**11**(3):241-248. DOI: 10.1109/TNSRE.2003.816873

[78] Barroso FO, Santos C, Moreno JC. Influence of the robotic exoskeleton Lokomat on the control of human gait: An electromyographic and kinematic analysis. In: 2013 IEEE 3rd Portuguese Meeting in Bioengineering (ENBENG). 2013. DOI: 10.1109/ENBENG.2013.6518442

Chapter 7

Transplantation or Transference of Cultured Cells as a Treatment for Spinal Cord Injury

Roxana Rodríguez-Barrera, Karla Soria-Zavala, Julián García-Sánchez, Lisset Karina Navarro-Torres, Estefanía de la Cruz Castillo and Elisa García-Vences

Abstract

Spinal cord injury (SCI) involves damage to the spinal cord causing both structural and functional changes, which can lead to temporary or permanent alterations. Even though there have been many advances in its treatment, the results of clinical trials suggest that the current therapies are not sufficiently effective. Recently, there has been a lot of interest in regulating this harmful environment by transplanting cultured cells and boosting their antiinflammatory cytokines and growth factors production. Several types of cells have been studied for SCI therapy including, Schwann cells (SC's), olfactory ensheathing cells (OECs), choroid plexus epithelial cells (CPECs), and immune cells (ICs) (lymphocytes, dendritic cells and alternative macrophage and microglia phenotypes). These treatments have shown to be promising and in this chapter, we will review the general aspects of transplanting these cells for SCI therapy as well as the neuroprotective and regenerative responses that different types of cells have reached in different SCI models. The mesenchymal stem cells (MSC) are one of the most well studied cell types; however, they were not included in this section because they will be reviewed in another chapter of this book.

Keywords: spinal cord injury, cultured cells, therapy

1. Introduction

SCI is a catastrophic condition that goes through two successive stages, which involves disturbances on ionic homeostasis, local edema, ischemia, focal hemorrhage, free radicals stress and inflammatory response [1]. SCI also causes partial or complete loss of sensory, motor and autonomic functions below the injury level, due to the interruption of the neural pathways. Nevertheless, cultured cells have successfully proved to achieve neuroprotective effects, by replacing or repairing damaged tissue, by neuronal survival, axonal growth, regulation of cytokine profiles and inflammation and motor recovery in animal models [2]. Cultured cells are promising strategies due to high variety of autologous cells that can be isolated and transplanted to patients; neural cells can up-regulate neurotrophic, growth and vascular factors to enhance the repair process in the spinal cord (SC). Also, non-neural cells can be polarized in vitro to evoke antiinflamatory responses in order to modulate SCI microenvironment. This still requires intensive investigation because cells from neural tissues such as OECs could only be retrieved by craniotomy with general anesthesia, which needs, optimized chirurgical practices and excellent preclinical and clinical cares [3]. However, mononuclear cells such as macrophages or lymphocytes isolated from peripheral blood, become a less invasive strategy [4, 5]. Although the current treatments for SCI have proven to have certain improvement effects, there is no actual cure for SCI [6]. That is why in recent years cell transplantation has become one of the most investigated approaches to treat this kind of disorder [7, 8].

2. Cultured cells

In this section, we will review each cell type separately because there are many differences and similarities among them which are worth mentioning.

2.1 Schwann cells

Numerous cell types have been studied and proposed for transplantation, however, SC's have always been considered as one of the best candidates for this treatment [9–11].

SC's are the principal glia of the peripheral nervous system (PNS) [12]. SC's wrap around long segments of peripheral nerves and produce myelin, forming a multilayered membranous sheath that allows axons to propagate action potentials at a high speed [12, 13]. The myelination of the axons by glial cells (oligodendrocytes in the central nervous system (CNS) and SC's in the PNS) is believed to be the last evolutionary step in the vertebrae nervous system and it's key in understanding neurophysiology [12, 14]. There are two types of SC's, the myelinating and non-myelinating both come from the neural crest cells in early development stages [15]. SC's precursors migrate along with growing axons in peripheral nerves where they receive specific signaling such as Neuregulin 1 (NRG 1) in order to survive and later on differentiate into myelinating SC's [15, 16].

SC's are essential for normal motor and cognitive functions, long-time integrity of the axons and they play a crucial role in axonal regeneration in the PNS after injury [6, 14, 17]. SC's regeneration role is more evident when you compare the outcome of a blunt injury in the SC with a similar injury in a peripheral nerve in rodents [18]. In several studies, it was seen that after sciatic nerve crush, the axons were able to rapidly grow back to their targets, also redundant myelin was removed and replaced with new myelin surrounding the regenerated axons, resulting in a generally normal tissue at an impressive speed (3–4 weeks) [14, 19]. On the other hand, crushing the SC results in the formation of a lesion filled with fluid or matrix leading to axonal retraction, permanency of myelin debris and absence of axonal regeneration [20]. In the PNS, the injury triggers a broad set of changes in the differentiation of both injured neurons and SC's, causing neurons to switch their function from cell to cell signaling to axonal growth and SC's change their function from axonal maintenance to support axonal regeneration [18, 21, 22]. This means that the glia in CNS does not suffer the same remarkable transformation as the PNS to repair the nervous tissue after the injury [19].

Those are some characteristic that have led them to become one of the biggest proposed treatments in cell transplants seeking to recover motor functions after SCI [9, 11].

2.1.1 Schwann cell response to injury

Even though axonal degeneration in the distal stump takes about 2–4 days, SC's response to axonal damage can be detected within hours of the injury, suggesting there is some communication between injured axons and SC's which needs further investigation [23]. As said before, right after de injury, SC's and undergo a large series of changes in gene expression to dedifferentiate into a non-myelinating immature type of SC's and proliferate extensively [24]. In this process myelin associated molecules such as the key myelin transcription factor Egr2 (Krox20), cholesterol synthesis enzymes, structural proteins, including P0, myelin basic protein (MBP), and membrane-associated proteins like myelin-associated glycoprotein (MAG) and periaxin are down-regulated, whereas molecules that characterize SC's in their immature stage (before myelination) are up-regulated [25]. These include L1, Neural cell adhesion molecule (NCAM), neurotrophin receptor p75NTR, and glial fibrillary acidic protein (GFAP) [24].

Another process in this response is the presence of phenotypes which are not associated neither with immature SCs nor with the SCs of an undamaged nerve. The appearance of these cells is critical, and since their main function is repairing, we refer to them as repair SC's or Bungner cells (BC's) [24]. The repair process includes, first, the up-regulation of neurotrophic factors such as, Glial cell-derived neurotrophic factor (GDNF), artemin, Brain-derived neurotrophic factor (BDNF), Neurotrophin-3 (NT3), Nerve growth factor (NGF), Vascular endothelial growth factor (VEGF), and pleiotrophin which promotes the survival of injured neurons and axonal regeneration [26]. Second, the BC's up-regulates the expression of inflammatory cytokines including tumor necrosis factor (TNF)-a, interleukin (IL)-1a,IL-1b, Leukemia inhibitory factor (LIF), and Monocyte chemoattractant protein-1 (MCP-1), in order to recruit macrophages that will eliminate redundant myelin that inhibit axonal growth [27].

2.1.2 Schwann cell transplantation in spinal cord injury

One of the first clues implicating that SC's transplantation could serve as a treatment for SCI was found in a set of experiments held by David and Aguayo in 1981. The experiments demonstrated that peripheral neurons (PN) lose their ability to regenerate over long distances in the PNS when they are submitted within the environment of a CNS graft and contrariwise the limited ability of CNS neurons to regenerate after an injury was enhanced within the environment of a PNS graft [19, 28]. Thanks to those landmark studies and decades of research, we now know that the introduction of SC's after a SCI can promote axonal regeneration, reduce tissue loss, and facilitate myelination of axons in order to improve sensory motor function [11, 29, 30].

One of the best-known mechanisms by which SC's promotes axonal regeneration is by the formation of bridges across the lesion site. The bridge is a multicellular structure that crosses the lesion rostrally to caudally, providing an environment in which axons can grow and also covering the glial scar which limits axonal regeneration [31]. Furthermore, the transplantation of SCs provides a neuroprotective effect preventing neuronal death from the continuous inflammatory reaction involved in the SCI [10, 11].

The PN-auto graft was one of the first techniques to promote axonal regeneration in the CNS after SCI. The nerve graft, besides providing supportive SCs it also endorses the survival of axotomized SC neurons by upregulating the expression of neuronal nitric oxide synthase (eNOS), furtherly activating the NO- dependent cyclic-GMP pathway, which enhances survival in these neurons [32, 33].

In addition, the PN-grafts promote the expression of growth factors in the host SC such as NGF and BDNF, delaying the formation of the glial scar, which is key for successful regeneration [34]. Another studied strategy is transplanting dissociated SCs alone into the injury. After transplantation, dissociated SCs are able to elicit axonal in-growth and align to secrete substrates, serving as guidance for axonal regeneration [35]. Moreover, when it comes to transplanting, the SCs alone have an advantage over the PN-graft, which is that purified SCs have the potential of being engineered to overexpress growth-promoting factors and/or adhesion molecules to enhance axon growth [36]. Even though several studies indicate that they cannot migrate into the host tissue, therefore regeneration outside the injury/graft site was limited [37].

However, their repair effect is not enough to induce an axonal response that leads to a full recovery of the locomotor function [38]. This could be due to the fact that a high percentage of SCs are lost in apoptotic or necrotic processes in the first 3 weeks after transplant [39]. This low survival rate post transplantation may be attributed to the prejudicial environment of the SCI in which low oxygen levels, inflammatory cytokines, reactive oxygen species (ROS) and cell-mediated immune reactions predominate [10, 39]. Also, after the injury reactive astrocytes, meningeal cells, and microglia form the glial scar which becomes a physical and chemical barrier for axons to grow. The glial scar induces the secretion of axonal growth and myelin-associated inhibitors such as chondroitin sulfate proteoglycans (CSPGs), semaphorins, and myelin-associated proteins which limits the regenerative capacity of SCs when transplanted alone [37]. This suggests that SC transplantation needs to be combined with additional interventions in order to ensure successful axonal regeneration and sufficient functional recovery after SCI [29].

Because of the multiple mechanisms and complex pathophysiology involved in SCI, a significant therapeutic effect on functional recovery may not occur with the transplantation of SCs alone, meaning that a combinational therapy strategy is most likely to be the best option [9]. There are many different strategies that have been studied and have shown to have beneficial results. First, the suspension of SCs in bioactive matrices promotes their survival and enhances their capacity for supporting axonal regeneration. Second, the complementary administration of neuroprotective agents, growth factors and other molecules improves the effects of SCs at the lesion site. Third, the inhibition of the glial scar formation and/or the reduction of its inhibitory cues to obtain axonal growth from grafts into the adjacent SC. Fourth, the co-transplantation of SCs with other cell types such as OECs, neural stem cells (NSCs), MSC and others. The different types of combinations as well as their characteristics and outcomes are described in **Table 1**.

The use of another cell population like OECs in the combinatory cell therapy had demonstrated to boost the SCs effects.

2.2 Olfactory ensheathing cells

OECs are a population of glia cells that are residents in the PNS and CNS, which are commonly located in the central olfactory bulb (OB) and the nasal olfactory mucosa (OM) [56]. They are accompanied by the envelope of olfactory nerve fibroblasts (ONFs), so they can embrace the bundles of olfactory nerve fibers from the nasal mucosa to allow the synapsis in the OB [57]. Recent studies have demonstrated that OB transplants could be differentiated to create relationships with the periphery and brain [56].

OECs express a lot of neurotrophic factors, including BDNF, GDNF, and NGF which are relevant for the propagations and guidance of axons, sharing properties with astrocytes and SC's [2]. Neurotrophic factors secreted by them is capable

	Outcome	Reference
Suspension matrices		
Matrigel (BD)	Significantly enhances long-term cell survival as well as graft vascularization and the amount of axonal ingrowth	[40]
PuraMatrix (BD)	Promotes their survival in the injured SC and reduces astrogliosis and locomotor impairment.	[41]
Alginic acid hydrogel	Reduces SC apoptosis and enhances recovery of locomotor function.	[42]
Growth factors and other molecules		
GDNF	Reduces astrogliosis and promotes axon regeneration, synapse formation, and locomotor recovery after SCI	[43, 44]
NRG1 + MSC	Reduce the size of cystic cavities, promotes axonal regeneration and locomotor recovery.	[45]
Rolipram + SCs grafts/ analog of cyclic AMP/ D15A	Promote significant supraspinal and proprioceptive axon sparing/regeneration and myelination. Promotes growth of serotonergic fibers into and beyond grafts, and significantly improves locomotion. Increases the size of SC grafts, the number of serotonergic fibers in the grafts, and the number of axons from the reticular formation below the lesion/implant.	[6] [6] [46]
Inhibition of the glial scar formation		
ChABC	Compared grafts treatment, it also improves forelimb and hindlimb movements as well as open-field locomotion. Decreases CSPGs both outside and within the SC transplant.	[47] [5, 48],
Polysialic acid	This leads to improved SC migration, axon regeneration, and locomotion.	[49, 50]
Combination cells		
MSC	Reduction of the size the size of cystic cavities, promotes axonal regeneration and locomotor recovery compared with SCs or MSC transplantation alone.	[45]
NSC	Promotes neuronal differentiation and functional recovery in after SCI in rats. Improves locomotion, increases axonal regeneration/ myelination, and reduces neuronal loss.	[51] [52, 53]
OECs	Regeneration of both proprio- and supra-spinal axons beyond the SC bridge. Significantly promotes axonal regeneration and improves locomotion.	[54] [55]

Table 1.
Combination of SCs transplantation with novel molecules/materials.

of protecting neurons, due to its faculty to inhibit scar formation and promote regeneration of axons (see **Table 2**) [58]. They also have an important ability in neural regeneration that consists in their proliferation and migration from PNS and CNS.

This attribute explains that enhancement of axonal extension after injury is possible and it can help neural regeneration, as a result of the expression of molecules implicated in that process (**Table 2**) [2, 59].

OECs phenotypes are different depending on their location in CNS or PNS. It has been shown that they express different types of molecules implicated in neuroregeneration, such as adhesion molecules, neurotrophic factors, proteases, cytokines and inhibitory factors.

Adhesion molecules	L1, E-NCAM, Laminin, Fibronectin, Type-V collagen
Neurotrophic (diffusible) factors/ receptors	NGF/p75, BDNF/TrkB, GDNF/GFRα-1, NTN/GFRα-2, NRG-1/ ErbB
Proteases (digest CSPG and PNN)	MMP2, MMP9, Serpine-1
Cytokines	IL-6/IL-6R, CX3CL1/Fractalkine, TGF-β3
Inhibitory factors/receptors	Nogo/NgR, Sema3A, EphrinA

Table 2.
OECs molecules implicated in neuroregeneration.

Otherwise, many studies have proved that OECs are capable of replacing apoptotic or necrotic neural cells, secreting numerous neurotrophins, and contributing to remyelination. Although they do not do the last function in the individual olfactory sensory axons, they enwrap abundant bundles of them, to assemble the nerve fascicles [60]. Recent findings have shown that neuroblasts recently generated in the subventricular zone, migrate into the OB [56].

2.2.1 Olfactory ensheating cells in response to injury

Studies showed that OECs have a significant therapeutic importance because they [47] interact with astrocytes from the CNS and establish connections with the second neurons. They have the aptitude to guide transected axons of the corticospinal tract throughout the focus of injury that causes the restoration of paw movements, supraspinal control of breathing and improvements in climbing after transplantation into high cervical SC injuries [47, 60].

It is well known that the SC enclose the long motor tracts descending from the brain and the long sensory tracts ascending to the brain. Therefore, it is essential to reconstruct them, and if it is not possible, it is necessary to at least establish a new circuitry with the ability to provide access to the information which was cut off by the injury [61].

2.2.2 Olfactory ensheating cells transplantation in spinal cord injury

Studies showed that OECs have a significant therapeutic importance because they interact with astrocytes from the CNS and establish connections with the second neurons. The implantation of these cells into the injured SC can intensify neurite growths into the distal part, promoting functional recovery. They have the aptitude to guide transected axons of the corticospinal tract throughout the focus of injury which causes the restoration of paw movements, supraspinal control of breathing, bladder and improvements in climbing after transplantation into high cervical SC injuries [55, 60, 62, 63]. Likewise, OECs transplanted from rats, dogs, pigs and humans into the lesion site in the SC of the rat, promote remyelination of injured axons and restore impulse conduction [48].

In normal conditions, OECs do not form myelin, but when are transplanted into the demyelinated SC, they have the capacity to form a peripheral pattern of myelin reminiscent of SC's myelin [40] There is also evidence that they reduce proteoglycans expression in reactive astrocytes after the injury [63]. Otherwise, microenvironment and culture conditions have an important influence on OECs behaviors in vitro and in vivo [41].

It has been demonstrated that OECs transplants can reduce posttraumatic cavity size, increase the sprouting of neurofilaments and serotonin axons, improve functionality and have neuroprotective effects [42, 64]. Due to these facts, several studies have ranked these cells as the second most commonly used cell type after SCI.

Recent studies have investigated the effect of co-transplantation of OECs and SCs at the injured site 7 days after contusion, demonstrating they significantly reduce the number of astrocytes, microglia/macrophage infiltration, and expression of chemokines (CCL2 and CCL3) at the injured site. These results suggest that OECs and SC's co-transplantation can promote the change of the macrophage phenotype from M1 secreting IFN-γ, to M2 secreting IL-4. The induction to M2 reduces ICs infiltration in the damaged site, regulates inflammatory factors and chemokine expression, which provide ICs environment for SCI repair [65].

2.3 Choroid plexus epithelial cells

The Choroid Plexus (CP) has a relatively simple structure. They consist of single layer of cuboidal to low cylindrical epithelial cells that reside on a basement membrane [43]. The main function is to form the cerebrospinal fluid (CSF). Approximately two thirds of this CSF is produced and secreted by the CP, the remainder produced by other areas such as the ependymal cells (ECs) of the ventricular surface and those cells lining the subarachnoid space. This fluid circulates in the ventricular system, subarachnoid spaces and spinal canal [44]. The CP, is not only implicate in CSF production also is a physical barrier to impede entrance of toxic metabolites to the brain [45]. Besides maintaining CNS homeostasis, CP and CSF have proven to be present in repairing processes after disease or damage [44].

The CP is located in the ventricular system of the brain. The ventricles consists of epithelial tissue which is highly vascularized by fenestrated blood vessels [46, 66]. Within the lateral ventricles, it propels from the choroidal fissure and extends from the interventricular foramen to the end of the temporal horn. It projects into the third and fourth ventricles from the ventricular roof. Grossly, the CP is lobulated with a single continuous layer of cells derived from the ependymal lining of the ventricles. Despite it, these cells possess epithelial cell characteristics and are often referred to as CP epithelial cells (CPECs) [66].

CPECs are the prolongation of ECs of the ventricular wall, and the underlying connective tissue corresponds to the pia mater covering the brain surface. CPECs and ECs are of ectodermal origin and develop from the neuroepithelium in the roof plate [49]. However, unlike ECs, CPECs are directly attached via basal laminae to the connective tissue, a feature characteristic of general epithelial cells pertain to a small group of polarized cells, where the Na-K-ATPase is expressed in the luminal membrane [50]. Ultrastructurally, the CPECs contain numerous mitochondria needed to maintain their metabolic work capability for both secretory activities and maintaining ionic gradients across blood-CSF barriers [54]. Underlying the epithelial cells and basal lamina is a dense vascular bed that provides a blood flow four to seven times greater than the rest of the brain [54]. Elsewhere, the cells have tight junctions closest to the luminal membrane to separate the ventricle lumen from the lateral intercellular and basal spaces. Adherence junctions are situated below the tight junctions, and desmosomes appear further below the adherence junctions [67]. The luminal surface is characterized by microvilli, both primary cilia and motile cilia [43]. The capillaries are large with thin fenestrated endothelial walls and bridging diaphragms overlying the fenestrations. An extensive array of adrenergic, cholinergic, peptidergic and serotoninergic nerve fibers innervate the blood vessels and the epithelium [67]. In addition, CP secrete many trophic factors such as Hepatocyte Growth Factor (HGF), Basic fibroblast growth factor (bFGF), insulin-like growth factor-II (IGF-II), NGF, and Transforming growth factor (TGF) [68].

CP recently have been recognized as an important immunological compartment in maintaining and restoring brain homeostasis. It has been reported that the CP is the primary gate for trafficking ICs from the vascular system to the CSF in CNS impairment [69]. In the healthy brain, T lymphocytes are mainly found at the CSF or at the "borders" of the CNS: the CP at the brain's ventricles, and the meningeal membranes that cover the brain [69].

2.3.1 Choroid plexus epithelial cells in response to injury

The evidence that the CP can instantly respond to signals coming from either the CNS itself or circulating immunity, suggests the possibility of controlling brain plasticity by affecting CP function [69], and identifies the cultured cells like CPECs as a novel target for neuroinflammatory conditions may involve a common underlying mechanism of CP immunomodulation.

CSF recirculation within the CNS happens through numerous various pathways. Recent revelations about a previously unappreciated meningeal lymphatic system of the CNS [51, 52]. Although ICs (excluding microglia) have no access to the brain parenchyma under homeostatic conditions, the meninges around the brain are populated by a lot of immune-cell types, which not only provide immune surveillance but also affect brain function [53].

T lymphocytes and their cytokines not only do harm but may also display homeostasis-restoring functions in the CNS [70]. ICs are also found within the CP epithelium, and during inflammatory events their numbers increase [71, 72], giving rise to the hypothesis that the CP is one of the points of immune-cell entry into the CSF [73].

2.3.2 Choroid plexus epithelial cells transplantation in spinal cord injury

When was examined the role of the CPCEs on inflammation after acute SCI: IL-1β, TNF-α, and hsp70 proved that the CPCEs may serve as an important source of these inflammatory mediators after SCI. There was also an inverse correlation between IL-1β and hsp70 staining and duration of clinical signs in acute SCI, suggesting that the expression increasing of these proteins by the CPECs could be of particular importance in the immediate-early inflammatory response after acute SCI [52].

Certain studies with CPECs showed that they are capable of promoting neurite extension as well as neuronal survival in vitro: in coculture with CPECs, neurons derived from the dorsal root ganglia or hippocampus presented extensions of long numerous neurites with elaborated branches on the surface of CPECs [74, 75].

Researcher indicating that CPCEs can promote nerve regeneration when grafted into SC lesions, the outcomes indicate by electron microscopy and immunofluorescence that CPECs labelling with green fluorescent protein (GFP) before transplantation closely interacted with growing axons, serving to support the massive growth of regenerating axons. Also, in this study Horseradish peroxidase (HRP) injection at the sciatic nerve showed that many HRP-labeled regenerating fibers from the fasciculus gracilis (FG) elongated into the graft 7 days after grafting. Furthermore, these regenerating axons from the FC were preserved for at least 10 months, with some axons elongating rostrally into the dorsal funiculus [76]. Recently, a study on CPECs transplantation, in which cultured CPECs were directly injected into the SC lesion, engrafted CPECs were located in the astrocyte devoid areas of the SCI; these data suggest that in rat, during the process of cavitation, reactive astrocytes may be reducted. In adittion, GAP-43-positive axons were found at the border of the lesion 2 days after transplantation [50] . Other study demonstrated that transplantation of

CPECs and MSC promotes axonal regeneration and enhances locomotor improvements. Overall this evidence suggests that they do not survive long term after transplantation into the SC. These date propose that some neurotrophic factors are released from those transplants to accelerate axonal regeneration through the astrocyte-devoid area formed in the epicenter of the lesion [77].

2.4 Lymphocytes and dendritic cells

Lymphocytes and dendritic cells (DCs) are ICs that are found in many different tissues within the body and work together achieved immunosurveillance and host defense against infection and injury. DCs are professional antigen presenting cells (APC) that capture, process antigens to initiate immune responses and express lymphocyte co-stimulatory molecules not only for activating lymphocytes, but, tolerizing T lymphocytes to antigens [78]. Indeed, lymphocytes are the mediators of the adaptative response by focus release growth factors and cytokine to the target cell, but only an efficient host defense is achieved through coordination of complex signals between innate and adaptative ICs: interaction between APC such as DCs with antigen and T lymphocytes [79].

Lymphocytes and DCs are derived from a hematopoietic stem cell in the bone marrow (BM); however, after certain cytokine secretion and transcription factors (TFs) expression, a common myeloid progenitor and common lymphoid progenitor are developed [80]. The first one differentiates into monocytes and DCs phenotype ($CD8\alpha^+$) [81, 82], while the second one give rise to different lymphocytes subsets, and a small population of $CD8\alpha^-$ DCs. DCs can be classified into myeloid or conventional DCs and plasmacytoid DCs. On the on hand, conventional can be divided into nonlymphoid tissue resident and lymphoid tissue residents and are well known for having a superior antigen processing, presentation machinery and ability to prime naive T lymphocytes responses; while plasmacytoid DCs express low levels of major histocompatibility complex class II (MHC-II) and costimulatory molecules [83]. In the case of lymphocytes, the bone marrow is where B lymphocytes maturation take place, while T lymphocytes development is generated in the thymus, by positive and negative selection to prevent potentially autoimmune reactions; only lymphocytes whose receptors interact weakly with self-antigens, and express a large repertoire of receptors capable of responding to a unlimited variety of non-self structures receive survival signals and are capable of migrating into peripheral lymphoid tissues as αβ naïve T helper (Th), thymic regulatory T (Treg), ($CD4^+$), cytotoxic ($CD8^+$) T lymphocytes [84]. Also, a distinct lineage of T lymphocytes: natural killer and γδ T lymphocytes, which play role in initial host response and exhibit limited plasticity [79, 85].

2.4.1 T lymphocytes in response to injury

When traumatic insult is carried out, an immune response is triggered in order to contain the damaged tissue but avoiding a negative impact in the host. That is why a cellular response most be properly balance by regulatory T lymphocytes [86]. $CD8^+$ T lymphocytes can differentiate principally in to regulatory and cytotoxic subsets, like the one that takes out Tc1 through the IL-12 influence, Tc2 differentiation from IL-4 and IL-6 plus TGFB can develop Tc17 with low cytotoxic activity [87]. $CD4^+$ T lymphocytes can differentiate into many classified subsets according to their cytokine pattern TFs, except for Th1 and Th2 subsets discovered by Mosmann and Coffman in the 1980s; who found that clonal population from Th1 principally secret IFNy and IL-4 in the Th2 subset [88]. Since that, $CD4^+$ T lymphocytes have diversified into a great number: Th9, Th17, T follicular helper (Thf) lymphocytes, induced regulatory T (iTreg) lymphocytes and Th22. Each $CD4^+$ T lymphocytes subset can be defined by their capacity to sense specific cytokines and function to control pathogens, prevent immune pathologies and contain damage in trauma such as SCI [89].

2.4.1.1 Lymphocytes as double-edged sword in spinal cord injury

T lymphocytes the arrival of T lymphocytes is crucial for the development of an autoreactive response and parenchyma destruction, due to unique anatomo-physiology of CNS through the release of proinflammatory cytokine entailing to more axon and cell bodies demyelination [90–92]. During acute phase, SC expresses high amounts of Th1 phenotype which is mainly regulated by IL-2, IL-12 and IFNγ. Moreover, in subacute phases IL-4, IL-13, IL-10, IL-17 and IL-23 cytokines are found in plasma and spleen, indicating the presence of Th2, Treg and Th17 profiles as an inefficient compensatory mechanism [93, 94]. Accordingly to this, for the last 10 years experimental findings have shown that T lymphocytes are not just pathogenic but beneficial. Schwartz and coworkers suggested that T lymphocytes play an important role in plasticity and in injured CNS by a still debated mechanism termed "protective autoimmunity" which it established that under certain physiological circumstances, autoimmune T lymphocytes specific to myelin basic protein (MBP), mostly $CD4^+$ can exert positive effect by protecting injured neurons [95].

2.4.1.2 Lymphocyte transferring after SCI

Lymphocytes that play complex role in SCI after antigen priming; the epitopes from neural proteins, can be considered beneficial, and Tregs can secret growth factors, shown neurotrophic factor receptors and promote progenitor differentiation and remyelination in damaged CNS [36, 96], authors have proposed T lymphocytes against MBP transfer as a therapeutic approach after SCI [97]. However, the only limiting factors are that in order to have a positive response, a genetic background and permissive microenvironment must be needed; susceptible individuals or strains don't possess control mechanism such as appropriate antigen presentation, ability to evoke regulatory T lymphocytes and neuroendocrine effect on ICs regulation [4, 98, 99]. Yoles and cols proved that T lymphocytes evoke a neuroprotective response after injury when animals that received T lymphocytes against MBP from injured animals improves hindlimbs locomotor activity, recovery from optic nerve injury, and mostly evoke an anti-inflammatory cytokine profile in the SC, suggesting that a physiological and beneficial response is developed after trauma [100]. In addition, it has been corroborated in different studies; IL-4-deficient animals enhance neuronal survival and increase functional after trauma when $CD4^+$ T lymphocytes from wild-type mice are transferred, but not from IL-4-deficient mice.

Inclusive, adoptive transfer of producing- IL-4, IL-10 and IL-3 CNS activated lymphocytes balance local inflammatory microenvironment by increasing protective cell populations like $CD4^+/Foxp3^+$ and $CD68^+/Arg1^+$ cells and in situ, proving that an increment of Th2 subset is beneficial to CNS repair [97, 101, 102]. But, increasing Treg population most be taking in consideration, due to injection of Treg can increase suppressive functions and limit effector T lymphocytes, which is negative to injured tissue in an optic nerve injury model [103]. Also, other studies proposed that Th1 profile is necessary for neuroprotection in SCI model [104], but not Th2 neither Th17. Only mice with Th1-conditioned cell transfer show motor recovery and present axon arbors extending from the main corticoespinal tract into the gray matter rostral to the lesion site; however, T lymphocytes were never primed with an specific antigen, or isolated from immunized animals [105].

In addition, to boost the restorative response, and reduce the risk of developing an autoimmune disease neural modified peptide (NMP) has been tasted by active and passive immunization. A91 is a peptide derived from an encephalitogenic epitope, amino acids 87–99 of MBP, by replacing the lysine residue 91 with alanine, which has evidence neural tissue preservation and paralysis reduction in rat model [106–109]. Also, passive p472 (Nogo-A derived peptide) immunization, promotes a T lymphocytes neuroprotective response, and no significant IgM antibody response, revealing that the design of this therapeutic cell strategies does not depend on humoral response and reduce the possibility of promoting clinical changes in CNS, like myelin oligodendrocyte glycoprotein in resistant and non-resistant strains [107, 110, 111].

2.4.2 Pulsed dendritic cells in spinal cord injury

Other studies support the idea that T lymphocytes response can be controlled from APCs transplantation into the traumatized mice and in non-human primates. Perhaps, APC must be primed first with NMP or SC homogenate (SHC), because, even mature DCs can evoke antigen-specific T lymphocyte response, it is not efficient enough to promote motor recovery [112]. Studies support the idea that only pulsed DCs can influence the secretion of neurotrophic factors like BDNF and neurotrophin-3 (NT3) in culture supernatants and at the SC lesion site via $CD4^{+}$T lymphocyte, motoneuron survival, NSCs proliferation and functional recovery [113–115]. Also, A91 has been used to pulse DCs, proving that motor recovery increase since the eleven days in comparison with control rats and an autoimmune response is not developed when Lewis strain is used but apparently a T lymphocyte response is involved, because when neonatally thymectomized rats are injected DCs treatment has no effect on recovery [116]. Furthermore, to promote regeneration, genetically modified fibroblasts to express BDNF have been tasted too. Cell therapy avoids secondary damage such as bleeding or infection that can be caused by growth factors or cytokine delivery in the site of injury [117].

2.4.2.1 Macrophage vs. microglia

In the early 1990s, macrophages and microglia were thought to arise from the same myeloid progenitor cell [118], however multiple sophisticated methods have discarded the bone marrow origin hypothesis, and it is proposed that microglia derives from primitive myeloid precursors that arise in the yolk sac early during embryonic development, maintaining it apart from the rest myeloid lineage [119]. Moreover, it was proved that Tgfb is needed for its differentiation in comparison with other myeloid cells [120], implicating, ontogenically, that microglia are not resident macrophages but, the authentic sentinels of CNS. In healthy CNS and during early post-natal period, microglia possess a resting phenotype with round and ameboid characteristics [121] however, lately, microglia develops into a ramified phenotype, which is equipped to keep CNS homeostasis in the developing and adulthood brain by phagocytic properties, trophic factors release for developing neurons and guidance of new vasculature [122]. Also, to keep a steady state, microglia maintains interaction between neurons by fraktalkine (CXCL1) and CD200 receptors to control inflammatory response and cell death [123, 124].

In respect of macrophage participation in CNS, it seems to be from monocytes which migrate from different sites during embryogenesis and in the adulthood [125]. Nevertheless, mostly are present in normal CSF [118], which contains about 5×10^{5} ICs in blood ratio of 1:2000 for monocytes (23%) [119]. Then, macrophages reside in the perivascular space, meninges and within the stromal matrix of CP, but not in neural parenchyma [126]. So, their principal function is the CNS immunosurveillance, that means, macrophages are one of the first APCs in interacting with antigens and T lymphocytes located in CFS, meninges and subarachnoid space, and thus, quickly phagocyte it or also optimize T lymphocytes reactivation and evoke a deleterious response such as autoimmune disease [127].

2.5 Alternative macrophage and microglia

Macrophages and microglia are both APCs that can be found in CNS under different functional phenotypes depending on the microenvironmental signals they received. In inflammation, microglia and macrophages express morphological changes, upregulate different cell markers and transcription factors. Microglia acquires a shape with shorter and thicker processes, increases CD45 expression and molecules for antigen presentation like MHCII, CD80 and CD86; also some miRNAs are related [128]. However, it is well known that activated macrophages and microglia can encompass two different functions. The first one is the classically activated M1 phenotype that is induced by IFNy or TNFa and secretes 1 l-12 and reactive oxygen intermediates. And the second one is an alternative subtype triggered by IL-4 and IL-13 cytokines and secretes TGFb and express arginase 1 [129]. To date, is not well stablished the appropriate cell markers to differentiate activated microglia from macrophages in CNS, but some populations have been proposed to differentiate the alternative phenotypes in monocytes: C3XCR1lo CCR2hi LY6Chi correspond to an inflammatory phenotype, while CX3CR1hi CCR2lo LY6Clo is found in the tissue remodeling phenotype [130, 131] and it has been corroborated in SCI studies; Shechter and cols. Proved that alternative M2 macrophages (Ly6cloCX3CR1hi) derived from monocytes traffic through CSF to provide an inflammatory response in SC [132].

Due to the important role that macrophages can play, several immunomodulatory therapies have been developed to control CNS response to pathological insults [123].

2.5.1 Macrophage and microglia in response to injury

Typically, damage stimulus triggers the activation of the microglia provoking the secretion of several cytokines like interferon gamma-induced protein 10, C-C motif chemokine ligand 1 (CCL1), C-C motif chemokine ligand 2 (CCL2) and C-C motif chemokine ligand 5 (CCL5) which recruit peripheral cells like macrophages. Microglia also participates in the adaptive immune response through the precise chemoattraction of T lymphocytes demonstrated in studies where the inhibition or stimulation of the resident microglia population resulted in abnormal recruitment [133].

These cells are considered essential screening damage monitoring constantly the microenvironment. Another important cell subgroup is the perivascular microglia which is replaced during 3 month period from bone marrow; its function is safeguarding the blood-brain barrier (BBB) through the recruitment of activated cell to BBB and parenchyma [134, 135].

2.5.2 Macrophage and microglia trafficking in response to injury

After a SCI take place an uncontrolled immune response that depends on the severity, level and mechanism of injury [136]. This cascade processes are characterized by pro-inflammatory and antiinflammatory alternatively activated cells [135]. The activation of phenotype M1 provokes neurotoxicity while type M2 promotes

Therapy	Treatment outcome	Reference
Adoptive transfer of M2 in rats	M2 phenotype reduces inflammation by increasing the number of $CD4^+$ $GATA3^+$ Th2 cells in the injured SC.	[144]
Incubated autologous macrophages in complete SCI: Phase I study	The study provides a preliminary evidence of safety and electrophysiological results. Also some patients present beneficial effects showing the efficacy of cell therapy.	[145]
Autologous macrophages delivery in patients with SCI	The clinical trial can be implemented in patients, however many factors contribute to a funnel effect in the study.	[5]
Azithromycin (AZM)	Increase M2 activation. Decrease M1 macrophage gene expression and potentiate M2 macrophage gene expression. Also, potentiate microglia vs. monocyte derived M2 macrophage activation. AZM improved locomotor function and coordination of mice recovering.	[146]
Anti- IL6-receptor (MR16–1 Ab)	Increased the area of spared myelin. Promoted functional recovery by promoting the formation of alternatively activated M2 macrophages.	[143]
Activated cultured microglia	Reduce the size of liquefaction necrosis area. Activated antiinflammatory mechanisms. Promote the hind limb motor function recovery.	[147]
Microglia/Macrophages activated with IL-1	Decrease of IL-1 participates in both the classical and alternative activation of microglia.	[148]
Recruitment of M2 macrophages	CP provide a route of macrophages derived monocyte (Ly6cloCX3CR1hi) to entry into the CNS to evoke an inflammatory response.	[132]

Table 3.
Immunomodulatory strategies for the microglia/macrophages response.

axon growth and remyelination [137]. This lead the efforts to develop immunomodulatory therapies to modify phenotypic and functional properties.

The activation of the glia occurs the first 24 hours after trauma [138]; while the peripheral monocytes migrate into the injury within the following 2 or 3 days post-injury, then they differentiate into macrophages that become phenotypically and morphologically indistinguishable [139].

The proinflammatory M1 macrophages vary along early stages releasing high levels of ROS to increase phagocytosis and cell recruitment removing foreign microbes and wound debris [140]; meanwhile M2 macrophages have some tissue repair properties through the release of immunosuppressive cytokines like IL-10 and C-C motif chemokines ligand 17, 18 and 22 to attract antiinflammatory leucocytes that increase the phagocytic receptors and upregulate growth factors [141].

There are three important chronological stages in the inflammatory response: the inflammatory, proliferative and remodeling phase and each one is characterized by certain cytokines and events. In the first one are present both M1 and M2a phenotypes, M1 secrete IL-1β, IL-12, TNF- α and IL-6 and M2a express high levels of IL-4, arginase-1 and Ym1 [142]. Comparative analysis of lesion development and intraspinal inflammation in four strains of mice following spinal contusion injury); during the second stage, keep going secreting proinflammatory cytokines but transition toward the expression of IL-10 and other antiinflammatory markers distinguished by the M2b macrophages followed by the M2c; in the third stage, the

M2c release high concentrations of IL-10, IGF1 [138]. Macrophage activation and its role in repair and pathology after SCI. TGF-β and a mannose receptor (CD206) with the decrease of arginase-1 and IL-12. At the end, the macrophages are deactivated and the inflammation resolves, this process can last several months. In brief, this sequence will provoke the axon dieback (classical macrophages) and remyelination, axon regeneration and the reduction of the dieback [143].

2.5.3 Macrophage and microglia in spinal cord injury

The manipulating macrophages facilitate maturation events typical of normal healing, for this reason it has been studied several methods to activate alternative macrophages and another strategy is better to improve the normal healing response by blocking certain pro-inflammatory mechanisms (**Table 3**).

3. Conclusions

The beneficial effects of cultured cells transplantation or transference in SCI have been demonstrated by numerous investigators and they are one of the main hopes for developing an effective treatment for SCI. This may be due to their great potential to amplify and genetically manipulate them in vitro, as well as all the complicated functions in axonal regeneration they possess. Furthermore, the development of cell transplantation derived from precursors show a higher ability to survive, integrate well with host tissue and support brainstem axon growth into and beyond the graft. However, the optimal source needs further investigation.

Recently, several clinical studies suggest their safety and feasibility, meaning that the transplantation of cultured cells have a significant therapeutic potential in persons with SCI. Nowadays, they are currently at an early stage of clinical testing following preclinical development.

Acknowledgements

We gratefully acknowledge to Universidad Anáhuac México Norte for your support to this project.

Author details

Roxana Rodríguez-Barrera, Karla Soria-Zavala, Julián García-Sánchez, Lisset Karina Navarro-Torres, Estefanía de la Cruz Castillo and Elisa García-Vences*
Centro de Investigación en Ciencias de la Salud (CICSA), Universidad Anáhuac México Campus Norte, Mexico

*Address all correspondence to: edna.garcia@anahuac.mx

References

[1] Zhou Y, Wang Z, Li J, Li X, Xiao J. Fibroblast growth factors in the management of spinal cord injury. Journal of Cellular and Molecular Medicine. 2018;**22**(1):25-37

[2] Gomez RM, Sanchez MY, Portela-Lomba M, Ghotme K, Barreto GE, Sierra J, et al. Cell therapy for spinal cord injury with olfactory ensheathing glia cells (OECs). Glia. 2018;**66**(7):1267-1301

[3] Tabakow P, Jarmundowicz W, Czapiga B, Fortuna W, Miedzybrodzki R, Czyz M, et al. Transplantation of autologous olfactory ensheathing cells in complete human spinal cord injury. Cell Transplantation. 2013;**22**(9):1591-1612

[4] Jones TB, Ankeny DP, Guan Z, McGaughy V, Fisher LC, Basso DM, et al. Passive or active immunization with myelin basic protein impairs neurological function and exacerbates neuropathology after spinal cord injury in rats. The Journal of Neuroscience. 2004;**24**(15):3752-3761

[5] Jones LA, Lammertse DP, Charlifue SB, Kirshblum SC, Apple DF, Ragnarsson KT, et al. A phase 2 autologous cellular therapy trial in patients with acute, complete spinal cord injury: Pragmatics, recruitment, and demographics. Spinal Cord. 2010;**48**(11):798-807

[6] Wang JM, Zeng YS, Wu JL, Li Y, Teng YD. Cograft of neural stem cells and schwann cells overexpressing TrkC and neurotrophin-3 respectively after rat spinal cord transection. Biomaterials. 2011;**32**(30):7454-7468

[7] Tsuji O, Miura K, Fujiyoshi K, Momoshima S, Nakamura M, Okano H. Cell therapy for spinal cord injury by neural stem/progenitor cells derived from iPS/ES cells. Neurotherapeutics. 2011;**8**(4):668-676

[8] Sahni V, Kessler JA. Stem cell therapies for spinal cord injury. Nature Reviews. Neurology. 2010;**6**(7):363-372

[9] Kanno H, Pearse DD, Ozawa H, Itoi E, Bunge MB. Schwann cell transplantation for spinal cord injury repair: Its significant therapeutic potential and prospectus. Reviews in the Neurosciences. 2015;**26**(2):121-128

[10] Pearse DD, Pereira FC, Marcillo AE, Bates ML, Berrocal YA, Filbin MT, et al. cAMP and Schwann cells promote axonal growth and functional recovery after spinal cord injury. Nature Medicine. 2004;**10**(6):610-616

[11] Takami T, Oudega M, Bates ML, Wood PM, Kleitman N, Bunge MB. Schwann cell but not olfactory ensheathing glia transplants improve hindlimb locomotor performance in the moderately contused adult rat thoracic spinal cord. The Journal of Neuroscience. 2002;**22**(15):6670-6681

[12] Nave KA. Myelination and support of axonal integrity by glia. Nature. 2010;**468**(7321):244-252

[13] Sherman DL, Brophy PJ. Mechanisms of axon ensheathment and myelin growth. Nature Reviews. Neuroscience. 2005;**6**(9):683-690

[14] Glenn TD, Talbot WS. Signals regulating myelination in peripheral nerves and the Schwann cell response to injury. Current Opinion in Neurobiology. 2013;**23**(6):1041-1048

[15] Jessen KR, Mirsky R. The origin and development of glial cells in peripheral nerves. Nature Reviews. Neuroscience. 2005;**6**(9):671-682

[16] Nave KA, Salzer JL. Axonal regulation of myelination by neuregulin 1. Current Opinion in Neurobiology. 2006;**16**(5):492-500

[17] Waxman SG. Axon-glia interactions: Building a smart nerve fiber. Current Biology. 1997;**7**(7):R406-R410

[18] Jessen KR, Mirsky R. The repair Schwann cell and its function in regenerating nerves. The Journal of Physiology. 2016;**594**(13):3521-3531

[19] Brosius Lutz A, Barres BA. Contrasting the glial response to axon injury in the central and peripheral nervous systems. Developmental Cell. 2014;**28**(1):7-17

[20] Dalamagkas K, Tsintou M, Seifalian A, Seifalian AM. Translational regenerative therapies for chronic spinal cord injury. International Journal of Molecular Sciences. 2018;**19**(6):1776

[21] Blesch A, Lu P, Tsukada S, Alto LT, Roet K, Coppola G, et al. Conditioning lesions before or after spinal cord injury recruit broad genetic mechanisms that sustain axonal regeneration: Superiority to camp-mediated effects. Experimental Neurology. 2012;**235**(1):162-173

[22] Barrette B, Hebert MA, Filali M, Lafortune K, Vallieres N, Gowing G, et al. Requirement of myeloid cells for axon regeneration. The Journal of Neuroscience. 2008;**28**(38):9363-9376

[23] Rotshenker S. Wallerian degeneration: The innate-immune response to traumatic nerve injury. Journal of Neuroinflammation. 2011;**8**:109

[24] Jessen KR, Mirsky R, Arthur-Farraj P. The role of cell plasticity in tissue repair: Adaptive cellular reprogramming. Developmental Cell. 2015;**34**(6):613-620

[25] Jessen KR, Mirsky R. Negative regulation of myelination: Relevance for development, injury, and demyelinating disease. Glia. 2008;**56**(14):1552-1565

[26] Brushart TM, Aspalter M, Griffin JW, Redett R, Hameed H, Zhou C, et al. Schwann cell phenotype is regulated by axon modality and central-peripheral location, and persists in vitro. Experimental Neurology. 2013;**247**:272-281

[27] Jessen KR, Mirsky R, Lloyd AC. Schwann cells: Development and role in nerve repair. Cold Spring Harbor Perspectives in Biology. 2015;**7**(7):a020487

[28] Aguayo AJ, David S, Bray GM. Influences of the glial environment on the elongation of axons after injury: Transplantation studies in adult rodents. The Journal of Experimental Biology. 1981;**95**:231-240

[29] Kanno H, Pressman Y, Moody A, Berg R, Muir EM, Rogers JH, et al. Combination of engineered Schwann cell grafts to secrete neurotrophin and chondroitinase promotes axonal regeneration and locomotion after spinal cord injury. The Journal of Neuroscience. 2014;**34**(5):1838-1855

[30] Pearse DD, Sanchez AR, Pereira FC, Andrade CM, Puzis R, Pressman Y, et al. Transplantation of Schwann cells and/or olfactory ensheathing glia into the contused spinal cord: Survival, migration, axon association, and functional recovery. Glia. 2007;**55**(9):976-1000

[31] Assinck P, Duncan GJ, Hilton BJ, Plemel JR, Tetzlaff W. Cell transplantation therapy for spinal cord injury. Nature Neuroscience. 2017;**20**(5):637-647

[32] Deng LX, Walker C, Xu XM. Schwann cell transplantation and descending propriospinal regeneration after spinal cord injury. Brain Research. 2015;**1619**:104-114

[33] Deng LX, Hu J, Liu N, Wang X, Smith GM, Wen X, et al. GDNF

modifies reactive astrogliosis allowing robust axonal regeneration through Schwann cell-seeded guidance channels after spinal cord injury. Experimental Neurology. 2011;**229**(2):238-250

[34] Kuo HS, Tsai MJ, Huang MC, Chiu CW, Tsai CY, Lee MJ, et al. Acid fibroblast growth factor and peripheral nerve grafts regulate Th2 cytokine expression, macrophage activation, polyamine synthesis, and neurotrophin expression in transected rat spinal cords. The Journal of Neuroscience. 2011;**31**(11):4137-4147

[35] Murray M, Fischer I. Transplantation and gene therapy: Combined approaches for repair of spinal cord injury. The Neuroscientist. 2001;**7**(1):28-41

[36] Dombrowski Y, O'Hagan T, Dittmer M, Penalva R, Mayoral SR, Bankhead P, et al. Regulatory T cells promote myelin regeneration in the central nervous system. Nature Neuroscience. 2017;**20**(5):674-680

[37] Oudega M, Xu XM. Schwann cell transplantation for repair of the adult spinal cord. Journal of Neurotrauma. 2006;**23**(3-4):453-467

[38] Fouad K, Schnell L, Bunge MB, Schwab ME, Liebscher T, Pearse DD. Combining Schwann cell bridges and olfactory-ensheathing glia grafts with chondroitinase promotes locomotor recovery after complete transection of the spinal cord. The Journal of Neuroscience. 2005;**25**(5):1169-1178

[39] Hill CE, Hurtado A, Blits B, Bahr BA, Wood PM, Bartlett Bunge M, et al. Early necrosis and apoptosis of Schwann cells transplanted into the injured rat spinal cord. The European Journal of Neuroscience. 2007;**26**(6):1433-1445

[40] Imaizumi T, Lankford KL, Kocsis JD. Transplantation of olfactory ensheathing cells or Schwann cells restores rapid and secure conduction across the transected spinal cord. Brain Research. 2000;**854**(1-2):70-78

[41] Mayeur A, Duclos C, Honore A, Gauberti M, Drouot L, do Rego JC, et al. Potential of olfactory ensheathing cells from different sources for spinal cord repair. PLoS One. 2013;**8**(4):e62860

[42] Lopez-Vales R, Fores J, Verdu E, Navarro X. Acute and delayed transplantation of olfactory ensheathing cells promote partial recovery after complete transection of the spinal cord. Neurobiology of Disease. 2006;**21**(1):57-68

[43] Damkier HH, Brown PD, Praetorius J. Cerebrospinal fluid secretion by the choroid plexus. Physiological Reviews. 2013;**93**(4):1847-1892

[44] Liddelow SA. Development of the choroid plexus and blood-CSF barrier. Frontiers in Neuroscience. 2015;**9**:32

[45] Schwartz M, Deczkowska A. Neurological disease as a failure of brain-immune crosstalk: The multiple faces of neuroinflammation. Trends in Immunology. 2016;**37**(10):668-679

[46] Johanson CE, Stopa EG, McMillan PN. The blood-cerebrospinal fluid barrier: Structure and functional significance. Methods in Molecular Biology. 2011;**686**:101-131

[47] Li Y, Decherchi P, Raisman G. Transplantation of olfactory ensheathing cells into spinal cord lesions restores breathing and climbing. The Journal of Neuroscience. 2003;**23**(3):727-731

[48] Vincent AJ, West AK, Chuah MI. Morphological and functional plasticity of olfactory ensheathing cells. Journal of Neurocytology. 2005;**34**(1-2):65-80

[49] Dziegielewska KM, Ek J, Habgood MD, Saunders NR. Development of the choroid plexus. Microscopy Research and Technique. 2001;**52**(1):5-20

[50] Kanekiyo K, Nakano N, Noda T, Yamada Y, Suzuki Y, Ohta M, et al. Transplantation of choroid plexus epithelial cells into contusion-injured spinal cord of rats. Restorative Neurology and Neuroscience. 2016;**34**(3):347-366

[51] Aspelund A, Antila S, Proulx ST, Karlsen TV, Karaman S, Detmar M, et al. A dural lymphatic vascular system that drains brain interstitial fluid and macromolecules. The Journal of Experimental Medicine. 2015;**212**(7):991-999

[52] Louveau A, Herz J, Alme MN, Salvador AF, Dong MQ, Viar KE, et al. CNS lymphatic drainage and neuroinflammation are regulated by meningeal lymphatic vasculature. Nature Neuroscience. 2018;**21**(10):1380-1391

[53] Kipnis J. Multifaceted interactions between adaptive immunity and the central nervous system. Science. 2016;**353**(6301):766-771

[54] Cornford EM, Varesi JB, Hyman S, Damian RT, Raleigh MJ. Mitochondrial content of choroid plexus epithelium. Experimental Brain Research. 1997;**116**(3):399-405

[55] Moore SA, Oglesbee MJ. Involvement of the choroid plexus in the inflammatory response after acute spinal cord injury in dogs: An immunohistochemical study. Veterinary Immunology and Immunopathology. 2012;**148**(3-4): 348-352

[56] Li L, Adnan H, Xu B, Wang J, Wang C, Li F, et al. Effects of transplantation of olfactory ensheathing cells in chronic spinal cord injury: A systematic review and meta-analysis. European Spine Journal. 2015;**24**(5):919-930

[57] Tabakow P, Raisman G, Fortuna W, Czyz M, Huber J, Li D, et al. Functional regeneration of supraspinal connections in a patient with transected spinal cord following transplantation of bulbar olfactory ensheathing cells with peripheral nerve bridging. Cell Transplantation. 2014;**23**(12):1631-1655

[58] Tang YY, Guo WX, Lu ZF, Cheng MH, Shen YX, Zhang YZ. Ginsenoside Rg1 promotes the migration of olfactory ensheathing cells via the PI3K/Akt pathway to repair rat spinal cord injury. Biological & Pharmaceutical Bulletin. 2017;**40**(10):1630-1637

[59] Anna Z, Katarzyna JW, Joanna C, Barczewska M, Joanna W, Wojciech M. Therapeutic potential of olfactory ensheathing cells and mesenchymal stem cells in spinal cord injuries. Stem Cells International. 2017;**2017**:3978595

[60] Ekberg JA, St John JA. Olfactory ensheathing cells for spinal cord repair: Crucial differences between subpopulations of the glia. Neural Regeneration Research. 2015;**10**(9):1395-1396

[61] Li Y, Li D, Raisman G. Interaction of olfactory ensheathing cells with astrocytes may be the key to repair of tract injuries in the spinal cord: The 'pathway hypothesis'. Journal of Neurocytology. 2005;**34**(3-5):343-351

[62] Woodhall E, West AK, Vickers JC, Chuah MI. Olfactory ensheathing cell phenotype following implantation in the lesioned spinal cord. Cellular and Molecular Life Sciences. 2003;**60**(10):2241-2253

[63] Wewetzer K, Verdu E, Angelov DN, Navarro X. Olfactory ensheathing glia and Schwann cells: Two of a kind? Cell and Tissue Research. 2002;**309**(3):337-345

[64] Wang S, Lu J, Li YA, Zhou H, Ni WF, Zhang XL, et al. Autologous olfactory lamina propria transplantation for chronic spinal cord injury: Three-year follow-up outcomes from a prospective double-blinded clinical trial. Cell Transplantation. 2016;**25**(1):141-157

[65] Zhang J, Chen H, Duan Z, Chen K, Liu Z, Zhang L, et al. The effects of co-transplantation of olfactory ensheathing cells and Schwann cells on local inflammation environment in the contused spinal cord of rats. Molecular Neurobiology. 2017;**54**(2):943-953

[66] Emerich DF, Skinner SJ, Borlongan CV, Vasconcellos AV, Thanos CG. The choroid plexus in the rise, fall and repair of the brain. BioEssays. 2005;**27**(3):262-274

[67] Praetorius J, Damkier HH. Transport across the choroid plexus epithelium. American Journal of Physiology. Cell Physiology. 2017;**312**(6):C673-C686

[68] Chodobski A, Szmydynger-Chodobska J. Choroid plexus: Target for polypeptides and site of their synthesis. Microscopy Research and Technique. 2001;**52**(1):65-82

[69] Baruch K, Schwartz M. CNS-specific T cells shape brain function via the choroid plexus. Brain, Behavior, and Immunity. 2013;**34**:11-16

[70] Ellwardt E, Walsh JT, Kipnis J, Zipp F. Understanding the role of T cells in CNS homeostasis. Trends in Immunology. 2016;**37**(2):154-165

[71] Giunti D, Borsellino G, Benelli R, Marchese M, Capello E, Valle MT, et al. Phenotypic and functional analysis of T cells homing into the CSF of subjects with inflammatory diseases of the CNS. Journal of Leukocyte Biology. 2003;**73**(5):584-590

[72] Young KG, Maclean S, Dudani R, Krishnan L, Sad S. $CD8^+$ T cells primed in the periphery provide time-bound immune-surveillance to the central nervous system. Journal of Immunology. 2011;**187**(3):1192-1200

[73] Marin IA, Kipnis J. Central nervous system: (Immunological) ivory tower or not? Neuropsychopharmacology. 2017;**42**(1):28-35

[74] Kimura K, Matsumoto N, Kitada M, Mizoguchi A, Ide C. Neurite outgrowth from hippocampal neurons is promoted by choroid plexus ependymal cells in vitro. Journal of Neurocytology. 2004;**33**(4):465-476

[75] Chakrabortty S, Kitada M, Matsumoto N, Taketomi M, Kimura K, Ide C. Choroid plexus ependymal cells enhance neurite outgrowth from dorsal root ganglion neurons in vitro. Journal of Neurocytology. 2000;**29**(10):707-717

[76] Ide C, Kitada M, Chakrabortty S, Taketomi M, Matsumoto N, Kikukawa S, et al. Grafting of choroid plexus ependymal cells promotes the growth of regenerating axons in the dorsal funiculus of rat spinal cord: A preliminary report. Experimental Neurology. 2001;**167**(2):242-251

[77] Ide C, Nakano N, Kanekiyo K. Cell transplantation for the treatment of spinal cord injury - bone marrow stromal cells and choroid plexus epithelial cells. Neural Regeneration Research. 2016;**11**(9):1385-1388

[78] Banchereau J, Steinman RM. Dendritic cells and the control of immunity. Nature. 1998;**392**(6673):245-252

[79] Charles A Janeway J, Travers P, Walport M, Shlomchik MJ. General properties of armed effector T cells. 2001;**8**:343-400

[80] Kondo M. Lymphoid and myeloid lineage commitment in multipotent

hematopoietic progenitors. Immunological Reviews. 2010;**238**(1):37-46

[81] Onai N, Obata-Onai A, Schmid MA, Manz MG. Flt3 in regulation of type I interferon-producing cell and dendritic cell development. Annals of the New York Academy of Sciences. 2007;**1106**:253-261

[82] Manz MG, Traver D, Miyamoto T, \Weissman IL, Akashi K. Dendritic cell potentials of early lymphoid and myeloid progenitors. Blood. 2001;**97**(11):3333-3341

[83] Merad M, Sathe P, Helft J, Miller J, Mortha A. The dendritic cell lineage: Ontogeny and function of dendritic cells and their subsets in the steady state and the inflamed setting. Annual Review of Immunology. 2013;**31**:563-604

[84] Charles A Janeway J, Travers P, Walport M, Shlomchik MJ. The development and survival of lymphocytes. 2001;7:258:342

[85] Jensen KDC, Su X, Shin S, Li L, Youssef S, Yamasaki S, et al. Lymphoid γδ T cells that develop in the absence of ligand produce IL-17 rapidly. Immunity. 2008;**29**(1):90-100

[86] Zhou L, Chong MM, Littman DR. Plasticity of $CD4^{+}$ T cell lineage differentiation. Immunity. 2009;**30**(5):646-655

[87] Huber M, Heink S, Grothe H, Guralnik A, Reinhard K, Elflein K, et al. A Th17-like developmental process leads to CD8(+) Tc17 cells with reduced cytotoxic activity. European Journal of Immunology. 2009;**39**(7):1716-1725

[88] Mosmann TR, Coffman RL. TH1 and TH2 cells: Different patterns of lymphokine secretion lead to different functional properties. Annual Review of Immunology. 1989;7:145-173

[89] DuPage M, Bluestone JA. Harnessing the plasticity of CD4(+) T cells to treat immune-mediated disease. Nature Reviews. Immunology. 2016;**16**(3):149-163

[90] Popovich PG, Wei P, Stokes BT. Cellular inflammatory response after spinal cord injury in Sprague-Dawley and Lewis rats. The Journal of Comparative Neurology. 1997;**377**(3):443-464

[91] Trivedi A, Olivas AD, Noble-Haeusslein LJ. Inflammation and spinal cord injury: Infiltrating leukocytes as determinants of injury and repair processes. Clinical Neuroscience Research. 2006;**6**(5):283-292

[92] Beck KD, Nguyen HX, Galvan MD, Salazar DL, Woodruff TM, Anderson AJ. Quantitative analysis of cellular inflammation after traumatic spinal cord injury: Evidence for a multiphasic inflammatory response in the acute to chronic environment. Brain. 2010;**133**:433-447

[93] Zong S, Zeng G, Fang Y, Peng J, Tao Y, Li K, et al. The role of IL-17 promotes spinal cord neuroinflammation via activation of the transcription factor STAT3 after spinal cord injury in the rat. Mediators of Inflammation. 2014;**2014**:2014:786947

[94] Mukhamedshina YO, Akhmetzyanova ER, Martynova EV, Khaiboullina SF, Galieva LR, Rizvanov AA. Systemic and local cytokine profile following spinal cord injury in rats: A multiplex analysis. Frontiers in Neurology. 2017;**8**:581

[95] Moalem G, Leibowitz-Amit R, Yoles E, Mor F, Cohen IR, Schwartz M. Autoimmune T cells protect neurons from secondary degeneration after central nervous system axotomy. Nature Medicine. 1999;**5**(1):49-55

[96] Ehrhard PB, Erb P, Graumann U, Otten U. Expression of nerve growth

factor and nerve growth factor receptor tyrosine kinase Trk in activated CD4-positive T-cell clones. Proceedings of the National Academy of Sciences of the United States of America. 1993;**90**(23):10984-10988

[97] Hauben E, Agranov E, Gothilf A, Nevo U, Cohen A, Smirnov I, et al. Posttraumatic therapeutic vaccination with modified myelin self-antigen prevents complete paralysis while avoiding autoimmune disease. The Journal of Clinical Investigation. 2001;**108**:591-599

[98] Kipnis J, Yoles E, Schori H, Hauben E, Shaked I, Schwartz M. Neuronal survival after CNS insult is determined by a genetically encoded autoimmune response. The Journal of Neuroscience. 2001;**21**(13):4564-4571

[99] Mestre H, Ramirez M, Garcia E, Martiñón S, Cruz Y, Campos MG, et al. Lewis, Fischer 344, and Sprague-Dawley rats display differences in lipid peroxidation, motor recovery, and rubrospinal tract preservation after spinal cord injury. Frontiers in Neurology. 2015;**6**:108

[100] Yoles E, Hauben E, Palgi O, Agranov E, Gothilf A, Cohen A, et al. Protective autoimmunity is a physiological response to CNS trauma. The Journal of Neuroscience. 2001;**21**(11):3740-3748

[101] Walsh JT, Hendrix S, Boato F, Smirnov I, Zheng J, Lukens JR, et al. MHCII-independent $CD4^+$ T cells protect injured CNS neurons via IL-4. 2015;**125**(6):2547

[102] Hu JG, Shi LL, Chen YJ, Xie XM, Zhang N, Zhu AY, et al. Differential effects of myelin basic protein-activated Th1 and Th2 cells on the local immune microenvironment of injured spinal cord. Experimental Neurology. 2016;**277**:190-201

[103] Walsh JT, Zheng J, Smirnov I, Lorenz U, Tung K, Kipnis J. Regulatory T cells in central nervous system injury: A double-edged sword. Journal of Immunology. 2014;**193**(10):5013-5022

[104] Kipnis J, Yoles E, Mizrahi T, Ben-Nur A, Schwartz M. Myelin specific Th1 cells are necessary for post-traumatic protective autoimmunity. Journal of Neuroimmunology. 2002;**130**(1):78-85

[105] Ishii H, Jin X, Ueno M, Tanabe S, Kubo T, Serada S, et al. Adoptive transfer of Th1-conditioned lymphocytes promotes axonal remodeling and functional recovery after spinal cord injury. Cell Death & Disease. 2012;**3**:e363

[106] Ibarra A, Hauben E, Butovsky O, Schwartz M. The therapeutic window after spinal cord injury can accommodate T cell-based vaccination and methylprednisolone in rats. The European Journal of Neuroscience. 2004;**19**(11):2984-2990

[107] Hauben E, Ibarra A, Mizrahi T, Barouch R, Agranov E, Schwartz M. Vaccination with a Nogo-A-derived peptide after incomplete spinal-cord injury promotes recovery via a T-cell-mediated neuroprotective response: Comparison with other myelin antigens. Proceedings of the National Academy of Sciences of the United States of America. 2001;**98**:15173-15178

[108] Martinon S, Garcia-Vences E, Toscano-Tejeida D, Flores-Romero A, Rodriguez-Barrera R, Ferrusquia M, et al. Long-term production of BDNF and NT-3 induced by A91-immunization after spinal cord injury. BMC Neuroscience. 2016;**17**(1):42

[109] Karin N, Mitchell DJ, Brocke S, Ling N, Steinman L. Reversal of experimental autoimmune encephalomyelitis by a soluble peptide variant of a myelin basic protein epitope: T cell receptor antagonism and

reduction of interferon gamma and tumor necrosis factor alpha production. The Journal of Experimental Medicine. 1994;**180**(6):2227-2237

[110] Stefferl A, Brehm U, Storch M, Lambracht-Washington D, Bourquin C, Wonigeit K, et al. Myelin oligodendrocyte glycoprotein induces experimental autoimmune encephalomyelitis in the "resistant" Brown Norway rat: Disease susceptibility is determined by MHC and MHC-linked effects on the B cell response. Journal of Immunology. 1999;**163**(1):40-49

[111] Wang L, Winnewisser J, Federle C, Jessberger G, Nave KA, Werner HB, et al. Epitope-specific tolerance modes differentially specify susceptibility to proteolipid protein-induced experimental autoimmune encephalomyelitis. Frontiers in Immunology. 2017;**8**:1511

[112] Wang Y, Wang K, Chao R, Li J, Zhou L, Ma J, et al. Neuroprotective effect of vaccination with autoantigen-pulsed dendritic cells after spinal cord injury. The Journal of Surgical Research. 2012;**176**(1):281-292

[113] Mikami Y et al. Implantation of dendritic cells in injured adult spinal cord results in activation of endogenous neural stem/progenitor cells leading to de novo neurogenesis and functional recovery. Journal of Neuroscience Research 2004;**76**(4):453-65

[114] Yaguchi M, Tabuse M, Ohta S, Ohkusu-Tsukada K, Takeuchi T, Yamane J, et al. Transplantation of dendritic cells promotes functional recovery from spinal cord injury in common marmoset. Neuroscience Research. 2009;**65**(4):384-392

[115] Wang K, Chao R, Guo Q-N, Liu M-Y, Liang H-P, Liu P, et al. Expressions of some neurotrophins and neurotrophic cytokines at site of spinal cord injury in mice after vaccination with dendritic cells pulsed with homogenate proteins. Neuroimmunomodulation. 2018;**20**(2):87-98

[116] Hauben E, Gothilf A, Cohen A, Butovsky O, Nevo U, Smirnov I, et al. Vaccination with dendritic cells pulsed with peptides of myelin basic protein promotes functional recovery from spinal cord injury. The Journal of Neuroscience. 2003;**23**(25):8808-8819

[117] Liu Y, Kim D, Himes BT, Chow SY, Schallert T, Murray M, et al. Transplants of fibroblasts genetically modified to express BDNF promote regeneration of adult rat rubrospinal axons and recovery of forelimb function. The Journal of Neuroscience. 1999;**19**(11):4370-4387

[118] Theele DP, Streit WJ. A chronicle of microglial ontogeny. Glia. 1993;**7**(1):5-8

[119] Greter M, Lelios I, Croxford AL. Microglia versus myeloid cell nomenclature during brain inflammation. Frontiers in Immunology. 2015;**6**:249

[120] Butovsky O, Jedrychowski MP, Moore CS, Cialic R, Lanser AJ, Gabriely G, et al. Identification of a unique TGF-beta-dependent molecular and functional signature in microglia. Nature Neuroscience. 2014;**17**(1):131-143

[121] Ling EA, Wong WC. The origin and nature of ramified and amoeboid microglia: A historical review and current concepts. Glia. 1993;**7**(1):9-18

[122] Kierdorf K, Prinz M. Microglia in steady state. 2017;**127**(9):3201-3209

[123] Cardona AE, Pioro EP, Sasse ME, Kostenko V, Cardona SM, Dijkstra IM, et al. Control of microglial neurotoxicity by the fractalkine receptor. Nature Neuroscience. 2006;**9**(7):917-924

[124] Hoek RM, Ruuls SR, Murphy CA, Wright GJ, Goddard R, Zurawski SM, et al. Down-regulation of the macrophage lineage through interaction with OX2 (CD200). Science. 2000;**290**(5497):1768-1771

[125] Guillemin GJ, Brew BJ. Microglia, macrophages, perivascular macrophages, and pericytes: A review of function and identification. Journal of Leukocyte Biology. 2004;**75**(3):388-397

[126] Bechmann I, Priller J, Kovac A, Bontert M, Wehner T, Klett FF, et al. Immune surveillance of mouse brain perivascular spaces by blood-borne macrophages. The European Journal of Neuroscience. 2001;**14**(10):1651-1658

[127] Kivisäkk P, Imitola J, Rasmussen S, Elyaman W, Zhu B, Ransohoff RM, et al. Localizing CNS immune surveillance: Meningeal APCs activate T cells during EAE. Annals of Neurology. 2009;**65**(4):457-469

[128] Ponomarev ED, Veremeyko T, Weiner HL. MicroRNAs are universal regulators of differentiation, activation, and polarization of microglia and macrophages in normal and diseased CNS. Glia. 2013;**61**(1):91-103

[129] Chazaud B. Macrophages: Supportive cells for tissue repair and regeneration. Immunobiology. 2014;**219**(3):172-178

[130] Shi C, Pamer EG. Monocyte recruitment during infection and inflammation. Nature Reviews. Immunology;**11**(11):762-774

[131] Geissmann F, Jung S, Littman DR. Blood monocytes consist of two principal subsets with distinct migratory properties. Immunity. 2003;**19**(1):71-82

[132] Shechter R, Miller O, Yovel G, Rosenzweig N, London A, Ruckh J, et al. Recruitment of beneficial M2 macrophages to injured spinal cord is orchestrated by remote brain choroid plexus. Immunity. 2013;**38**(3):555-569

[133] Mrass P, Weninger W. Immune cell migration as a means to control immune privilege: Lessons from the CNS and tumors. Immunological Reviews. 2006;**213**:195-212

[134] Hickey WF, Vass K, Lassmann H. Bone marrow-derived elements in the central nervous system: An immunohistochemical and ultrastructural survey of rat chimeras. Journal of Neuropathology and Experimental Neurology. 1992;**51**(3):246-256

[135] Stoll G, Jander S. The role of microglia and macrophages in the pathophysiology of the CNS. Progress in Neurobiology. 1999;**58**(3):233-247

[136] David S, Kroner A. Repertoire of microglial and macrophage responses after spinal cord injury. Nature Reviews. Neuroscience. 2011;**12**(7):388-399

[137] Shechter R, Schwartz M. Harnessing monocyte-derived macrophages to control central nervous system pathologies: No longer 'if' but 'how. The Journal of Pathology. 2013;**229**(2):332-346

[138] Gensel JC, Zhang B. Macrophage activation and its role in repair and pathology after spinal cord injury. Brain Research. 2015;**1619**:1-11

[139] Novak ML, Koh TJ. Phenotypic transitions of macrophages orchestrate tissue repair. The American Journal of Pathology. 2013;**183**(5):1352-1363

[140] Hall ED, Springer JE. Neuroprotection and acute spinal cord injury: A reappraisal. NeuroRx. 2004;**1**(1):80-100

[141] Gurtner GC, Werner S, Barrandon Y, Longaker MT. Wound

repair and regeneration. Nature. 2008;**453**(7193):314-321

[142] Kigerl KA, McGaughy VM, Popovich PG. Comparative analysis of lesion development and intraspinal inflammation in four strains of mice following spinal contusion injury. The Journal of Comparative Neurology. 2006;**494**(4):578-594

[143] Guerrero AR, Uchida K, Nakajima H, Watanabe S, Nakamura M, Johnson WE, et al. Blockade of interleukin-6 signaling inhibits the classic pathway and promotes an alternative pathway of macrophage activation after spinal cord injury in mice. Journal of Neuroinflammation. 2012;**9**:40

[144] Ma SF, Chen YJ, Zhang JX, Shen L, Wang R, Zhou JS, et al. Adoptive transfer of M2 macrophages promotes locomotor recovery in adult rats after spinal cord injury. Brain, Behavior, and Immunity. 2015;**45**:157-170

[145] Knoller N, Auerbach G, Fulga V, Zelig G, Attias J, Bakimer R, et al. Clinical experience using incubated autologous macrophages as a treatment for complete spinal cord injury: Phase I study results. Journal of Neurosurgery. Spine. 2005;**3**(3):173-181

[146] Zhang B, Bailey WM, Kopper TJ, Orr MB, Feola DJ, Gensel JC. Azithromycin drives alternative macrophage activation and improves recovery and tissue sparing in contusion spinal cord injury. Journal of Neuroinflammation. 2015;**12**:218

[147] Yu TB, Cheng YS, Zhao P, Kou DW, Sun K, Chen BH, et al. Immune therapy with cultured microglia grafting into the injured spinal cord promoting the recovery of rat's hind limb motor function. Chinese Journal of Traumatology. 2009;**12**(5):291-295

[148] Sato A, Ohtaki H, Tsumuraya T, Song D, Ohara K, Asano M, et al. Interleukin-1 participates in the classical and alternative activation of microglia/macrophages after spinal cord injury. Journal of Neuroinflammation. 2012;**9**:65

Chapter 8

Neuroregenerative-Rehabilitative Therapy for Spinal Cord Injury

Alok Sharma, Hemangi Sane, Nandini Gokulchandran, Prerna Badhe, Amruta Paranjape, Pooja Kulkarni and Vivek Nair

Abstract

Spinal cord injury is one of the leading causes of disability worldwide. Current mainstay treatment strategies consist of surgical and medical management in acute and subacute stage. Rehabilitative management in the chronic stage. None of the existing strategies can repair the damage to the spinal cord and recover neurological functioning. Stem cells have promising results in pre-clinical and clinical studies. Various pre-clinical studies have evidenced neuro-regenerative capabilities of stem cells and shown neural recovery. Clinical studies have also shown improvements in neurological functions and quality of life. This chapter discusses about different types of cells available, routes of administration available to transplant these cells, dosages of cell and optimum time after injury at which cells should be transplanted based on world-wide literature. We have also discussed results following our protocol of intrathecal transplantation of autologous bone marrow mononuclear cells. Although, not a cure, stem cell therapy further improves quality of life, functional independence and reduces secondary complications when combined with existing treatment strategies; neuroregenerative rehabilitative therapy.

Keywords: stem cell therapy, autologous, bone marrow mononuclear cells, spinal cord injury, paracrine effect, neurorestoration

1. Introduction

Spinal cord injury (SCI) is a disabling neurologic disorder that can lead to motor and sensory impairment causing, paraplegia or tetraplegia. It can also exhibit bladder and bowel impairment, respiratory impairment and autonomic dysfunction [1].

The incidence of the disease is estimated to be 223–755 per million worldwide [2, 3]. The healing and recovery process during different phases since the time of injury differ significantly [4].

Current treatment options consist of surgical management complimented by administration of methylprednisolone in the acute stage; prevention of secondary injury in the sub-acute stage and multidisciplinary rehabilitation management in the chronic stage. Due to insufficient neuroregenerative capabilities of these treatments, they fail to reverse the damage to neurons and symptoms of neurological deficit [5–8]. Therefore, there is an unmet medical need which warrants exploring novel neurorestorative strategies.

Stem cell therapy has emerged as a promising regimen to bring about neuroregeneration and neural functional benefits, hence can be termed as neuroregenerative therapy. Various cell types being explored for their effectiveness are bone mesenchymal stem cells (BMSCs), bone marrow mononuclear cells (BMMNCs), umbilical cord-derived mesenchymal stem cells (UCMSCs), adipose-derived stem cells (ADSCs), olfactory ensheathing cells (OECs), and fetal brain-derived neural stem/progenitor cell (FB-DNS/PCs), induced pluripotent stem cells (iPSCs) and others [9–12].

The earliest attempt in translational research were by Geron Corporation who had announced a clinical trial using human embryonic stem cell (ESC)-derived oligodendrocyte progenitor cells (OPCs) in patients with spinal cord injury at the site of the lesion [13]. Due to ethical and safety risks involved in ESC they were not widely accepted for clinical use. Advent of knowledge of the role of adult stem cells in natural repair processes of the body lead to clinical exploration of these cells. Some of the earliest published work was by Geffner et al. in 2008, by transplantation of adult bone marrow stem cells through multiple routes, that is, intraspinal, intrathecal and intravenous in patients with SCI [14]. The study demonstrated that these cells and routes were safe and feasible. Many adult stem cell types, routes and clinical protocols have since been tested clinically [14–33].

Clinical outcome and effectiveness of cell transplantation remains variable due to the heterogenicity of cell types, dosages, route of transplantation, level of manipulation and treatment regimens followed thereafter. This chapter provides a detail review about different stem cell therapies available for the management of spinal cord injury and their clinical outcomes as seen in published literature.

2. What are stem cells?

Stem cell is an undifferentiated cell, which can self-renew to replicate itself as well as give rise to the specialized cells under appropriate conditions [34].

Stem cells are the undifferentiated cells that can give rise to progeny identical to themselves (de-differentiation) or specialized cells different from them (trans-differentiation). All regenerative processes in the human body during developmental pre-natal stages as well as post-natal and adult stages follow these two routes. Recently, the technological advances have given rise to another route, reprogramming cells to acquire properties of trans-differentiation [35].

Depending upon their ability to de-differentiate or transdifferentiate, the source of cells, processing required to harvest the cells and host in which cells are transplanted; the cells can be categorized into various types which are described in detail in the next section.

3. Types of stem cells

3.1 Based on the potency of cells

Depending upon their differentiation potential, cells are classified as unipotent, multipotent, pluripotent and totipotent (**Figure 1**).

Totipotent cells can differentiate into embryonic as well as extraembryonic and placental cells [36]. Pluripotent cells can differentiate into embryonic cells only.

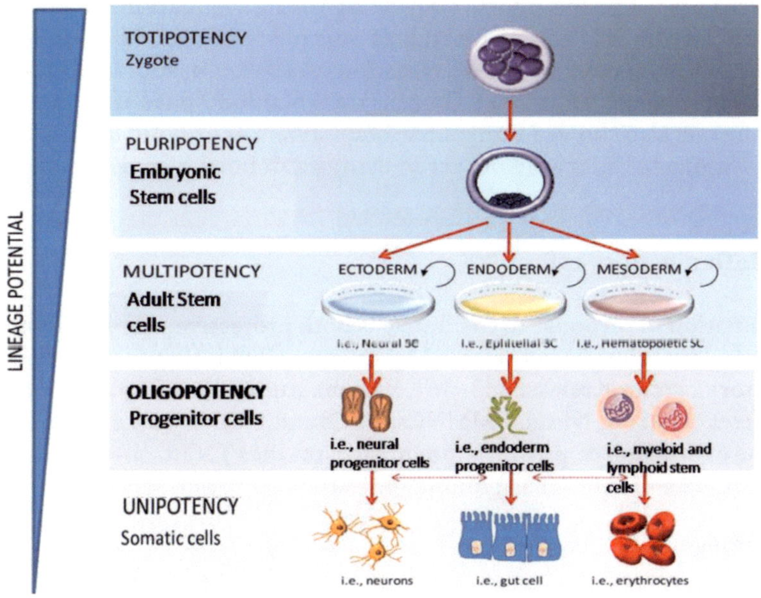

Figure 1.
Different types of cells based on their potency.

These possess the property of de-differentiation as well as trans-differentiation into cell types of all three germ layers [36]. Cells that can be harvested after birth are called 'adult stem cells'. Most of the adult stem cells are multipotent or unipotent. Multipotent cells possess the property of trans-differentiation into cells of different tissues whereas unipotent cells can only de-differentiate to create progeny identical to themselves or a differentiated cell type of only one specific tissue [37].

3.2 Based on the host in whom cells are transplanted

If the cells are harvested from and transplanted to the same person, these are called autologous cells; but if the cells are harvested from a host different from that of the recipient these are called allogenic cells.

4. Mechanism of action of stem cells in spinal cord injury

4.1 Remyelination

The immediate impact of injury to spinal cord is on the ascending and descending pathways and blood vessels in the spinal cord. Disrupted circulation leads to infarction of the local tissue due to hypoxia and ischemia causing neuronal loss and demyelination. This is clinically presented as spinal shock, systemic hypotension, vasospasm, ischemia, ionic imbalance and neurotransmitter accumulation [38]. Transplantation of cells can remyelinate damaged tissue and aid in symptom recovery. Human ESC-derived OPCs transplanted into the rats with spinal cord injury showed enhanced remyelination and locomotor ability when transplanted in the sub-acute phase as opposed to chronic phase after spinal cord injury [39]. Neural precursor cells also showed differentiation into oligodendrocytes ensheathing the axons, these cells expressed myelin suggesting the remyelination potential of these cells. Rat models, both in sub-acute and chronic phase of spinal cord injury showed improved functional outcome. Remyelination was better in sub-acute as compared with chronic phase [40]. Human UCB cells transplanted 7 days after spinal cord injury in the rats also showed remyelination of axons improving functional outcome [41]. Similar results were observed using adult bone marrow mononuclear cells [42].

4.2 Anti-inflammatory effect

Inflammation in response to the injury is both protective and damaging to the tissue. Secondary injury is perpetrated by uncontrolled inflammatory response pro-inflammatory cytokine release [43–46]. Various studies have explored anti-inflammatory effect of MSCs, NPCs, BMMNCs, ESCs and UCB cells. Cell transplantation reduces the expression of pro-inflammatory cytokines TNFα, IL-4, IL-1β, IL-2, IL-6, IL-7, IL-12 and interferon gamma [47–50].

4.3 Neoangiogenesis

Transplanted cells have been shown to secrete various growth factors and stimulate the resident cells to secret these factors through their paracrine effect. One of the growth factors secreted is vascular endothelial growth factor (VEGF) which stimulates neoangiogenesis. This proangiogenic effect has been evidenced by increased vascularization of the lesion area in various preclinical studies [51–54].

4.4 Neuro-regeneration

Transplanted cells of various cells possess neurogenic potential. Cells have been shown to differentiate into neuronal as well as non-neuronal tissues. Axon sprouting is noticed in the transplanted regions. Endogenous neurogenetic processes are also catalyzed by the growth factors like brain-derived neurotrophic factor (BDNF) secreted by these cells. Synaptic pruning is also observed. These changes are further reinforced by the functional locomotor recovery seen post transplantation [55, 56].

4.5 Neurotrophic and antiapoptotic effect

Cells secret and facilitate endogenous secretion of various growth factors like fibroblast growth factor (FGF), vascular endothelial growth factor (VEGF), neural growth factor (NGF), glial cell line-derived neurotrophic factor and brain-derived neurotrophic factor (BDNF). These wield neurotrophic effect protecting the neurons from secondary injury and apoptosis (**Figure 2**) [54, 57].

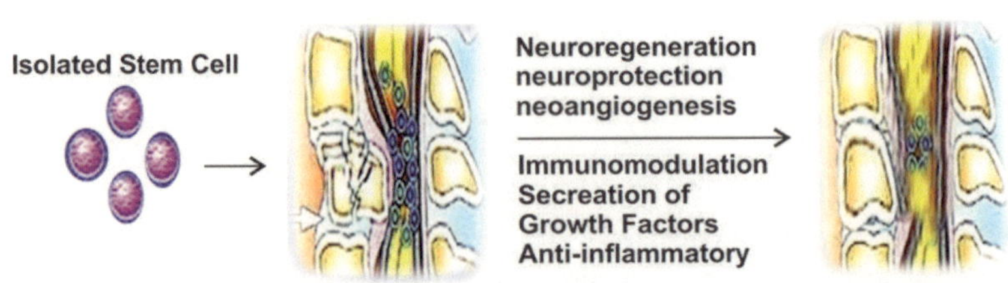

Figure 2.
Bone marrow aspiration.

5. Literature review of published evidence for efficacy of stem cells

5.1 Pre-clinical

5.1.1 Human embryonic stem cells (hESCs)

These cells can be harvested from preimplantation blastocyst after immunosurgical removal of trophectoderm to access the inner cells mass [58]. hESCs are pluripotent and can differentiate into cells of ectodermal origin, that is, neuronal and glial cells. hESCs derived oligodendrocyte progenitor cells (OPCs) have shown neuronal recovery more effectively in the acute phase as compared to chronic phase of spinal cord injury [39, 59, 60]. Neural stem cells (NSCs) have the potential to differentiate into neural and non-neural tissue. Neuroregenerative potential of these exhibited as remyelination of damaged axons and secretion of neurotrophic factors enhancing neuronal survival post SCI in mice [61–63].

Despite promising results in pre-clinical studies, clinical translation of these is limited due to ethical concerns, risk of immune rejection and tumorigenicity [64].

5.1.2 Multipotent stem cells

Adult stem cells like bone marrow stromal cells (BMSCs), mesenchymal stem cells (MSCs), umbilical cord stromal cells (UCSCs), umbilical cord mesenchymal cells (UC-MSCs), adipose-derived stem cells and dental pulp-derived stem cells are examples of multipotent stem cells [51]. MSCs and BMSCs are easy to harvest as they are available in the bone marrow. However, MSCs are available in a small number and therefore need to be expanded in-vitro before transplantation. These cells can migrate and home onto the site of injury therefore can be administered through a less invasive route distant from the site of injury. Unlike pluripotent cells, these cells show better functional recovery in chronic SCI [41, 42, 65]. Transplantation of these cells has shown functional and motor recovery in rats after SCI in several studies. These benefits are postulated to be due to neurotrophic, immunomodulatory and neoangiogenic effect of these cells in addition to their ability to differentiate neural cells [66].

5.1.3 Induced pluripotent stem cells (iPSCs)

Last decade has seen rise in efforts to develop technologies to improve quality and efficiency of reprogramming of cells to induce pluripotency. iPSCs are also pluripotent and give rise to neuronal as well as non-neuronal tissue. Transplantation of progenitors derived from iPSCs have shown ability for remyelination of damaged neurons and improved nerve conduction. These cells can migrate long distances and therefore can be administered at a remote site which is less invasive. Apart from neuroregeneration, the cells are also capable of immunomodulation and synaptic reconstruction [67–72].

The technology is still in its nascent stage, although promising, successful clinical translation has barriers.

5.2 Clinical

5.2.1 Embryonic stem cells (ESCs)

One of the earliest studies used cells from the fetal nervous and hemopoietic tissues in 15 SCI patients with no side effects [73]. However, due to various ethical and medical concerns the use of these cells in clinical trials and application is restricted worldwide.

5.2.2 Multipotent stem cells

Various studies have explored and demonstrated safety and feasibility of multipotent stem cells [15, 17, 74–83].

5.2.2.1 Bone marrow mononuclear cells

In a comparison between transplantation of autologous bone marrow cells directly into the SCI sites administered with subcutaneous injections of granulocyte macrophage colony stimulating factor (GM-CSF) {n = 5} and only administration of GM-CSF {n = 1}, combination group showed better improvements. Improvements were noted during 3–7 months post procedure, 1 patient from the combination group showed change in the AIS grade as well. There were mild side effects associated with GM-CSF administration like Fever, myalgia and leukocytosis; however, there were no irreversible adverse events noted, neither was there any neurological deterioration [16]. Kumar et al. studied the effect of bone marrow mononuclear cells and noted that there was perceptible improvement in 32.6% of the patients with no major irreversible adverse effects. Outcome did not vary with the time taken from the injury till intervention [35]. Al-Zoubi et al. demonstrated the positive effect of purified autologous leukapheresis-derived CD34+ and CD133+ stem cells in 19 cases of chronic SCI [29]. Our published results with mononuclear cells are discussed in detail in the later part of the chapter [84, 85].

5.2.2.2 Mesenchymal cells

In a novel method, using combination of bone marrow mesenchymal stem cells (BM-MSC) and patient's autoimmune T cells, Moviglia et al. demonstrated the neuro-regeneration phenomenon-based changes in the inflammatory processes at the site of injury. Both the patients showed motor and sensory recovery with no adverse effects [17]. Peripheral stem cells and macrophages have also been reported to show improvements of motor and sensory functions without any adverse effects [18, 19]. Cheng et al. in a controlled study including 34 cases of thoracolumbar spinal cord injury, stated that umbilical cord mesenchymal stem cells effectively improve neurological functional recovery after spinal cord injury, and its efficacy is superior to that of rehabilitation therapy and self-healing [30].

5.2.2.3 Others

Other sources such as cord blood, olfactory ensheathing cells and adipose tissue derived stem cells also showed improvement in sensory-motor functional improvements [20–24]. Saberi et al. studied the safety of intramedullary Schwann cell transplantation in 33 patients over the period of 2 years, there were no tumor formation or other adverse events recorded [25].

5.2.2.4 Co-transplantation of multiple cell types

Co-transplantation of cells has also been explored. Combined use of olfactory ensheathing cells and Schwann cells enhanced functional recovery [27]. Similarly,

Chen et al. in their study of 28 cases showed beneficial effects of OECs, SCs, or a combination of them in SCI [28].

Multipotent adult stem cells are safe to use clinically and have demonstrated improved neurological outcome.

5.2.3 Routes of transplantation

Several comparative studies have been carried out to determine the optimum route of administration. Geffner et al. reported administration of BMSCs intravenous, into the spinal canal and into the spinal cord to be safe and feasible. They also demonstrated improved ASIA, Barthel Index. Ashworth and Frenkel scores suggesting improved quality of life in most patients [14]. While intra-arterial transplantation of autologous bone marrow stem cells showed more improvements as compared with that of intravenous route, intravenous transplantation showed better neurological outcome as compared to the site of injury [31–33]. Systemic routes show considerable dilution of cells at various cells like kidneys, liver, spleen and lungs. Several intraspinal approaches like intraparenchymal, intralesional and intramedullary approaches have been explored. Although no serious adverse events were noted; some patients complained of transient increase in paresthesia and muscle cramps. Intraspinal approaches are associated with increased risk of procedure related adverse effect due to invasive nature of the procedure [86–88]. Saito et al. [89], Pal et al. [90] and Kumar et al. [91] reported intrathecal administration to be the optimum route of administration. Although in this approach cells are transplanted away from the lesion area, MRI studies of radiolabeled cells have shown successful homing of cells at the site of injury [92].

6. Published clinical results of NeuroGen Brain and Spine Institute

6.1 Our protocol

6.1.1 Pre-intervention protocol

All the patients are thoroughly assessed clinically to rule out presence of active infections, HIV or HBsAg positive status and malignancies. Routine serological tests and chest X-ray are performed to ensure medical fitness. Neuroimaging using functional MRI brain and MRI of spine is performed. Various clinical outcome measures are marked before procedure assessing muscle tone, strength, ambulation and sensations. Granulocyte colony stimulating factor injections are given 48 and 24 h prior to the transplantation to enhance proliferation of cells in the bone marrow.

6.1.2 Intervention protocol

Our protocol has been designed after careful review of available literature. The protocol for harvesting and transplanting the cells is minimally invasive with no major adverse effects. It consists of three steps.

6.1.2.1 Aspiration of bone marrow

80–120 ml of bone marrow is aspirated from anterior superior iliac spine (**Figure 3**).

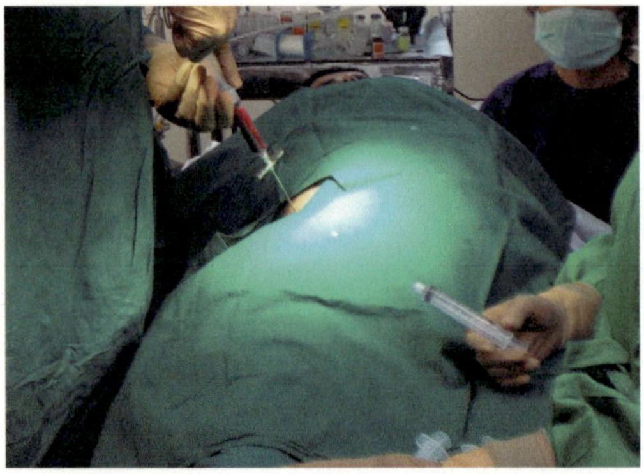

Figure 3.
Separation of BMMNCs.

6.1.2.2 Separation of BMMNCs

Density gradient method is used to separate the bone marrow mononuclear cell fraction which is then analyzed under microscope using Trypan blue to check for viability of the mononuclear cells. FACS analysis is used to identify CD34+ cells and viability, cell count and percentage of CD34+ cells are calculated (**Figure 4**).

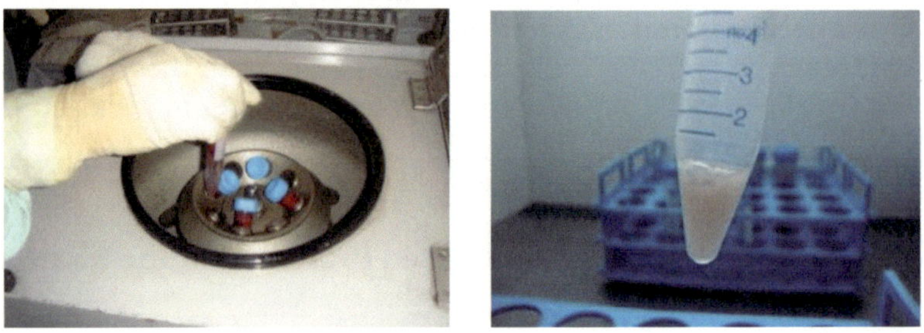

Figure 4.
Injection of BMMNCs.

6.1.2.3 Injection

Separated cell fraction is transplanted intrathecally in the space between L4 and L5 lumbar vertebrae by lumbar puncture. This is performed under local anesthesia and sterile conditions in the operation theatre (**Figure 5**).

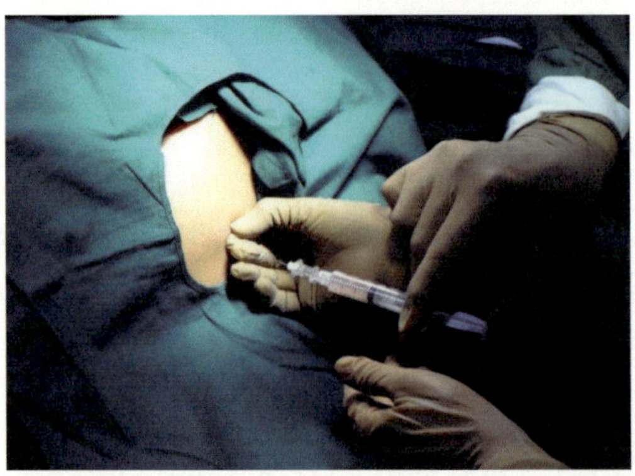

Figure 5.
Mechanism of action of stem cells for the treatment of spinal cord injury.

6.1.3 Post intervention protocol

After the cell transplantation a home program of rigorous rehabilitation is prescribed Many of the patients show deficiencies due to prolonged immobility and poor nutrition, therefore nutritional supplements are prescribed as and when required. Patients are regularly followed up every 3 months.

6.1.4 Rationale for the protocol

Autologous cells are used to reduce the risk of immune rejection. Bone marrow mononuclear cells (BMMNCs) fraction consists of various cells types including mesenchymal cells, hematopoietic progenitor cells, side population cells, stromal cells and very small embryonic like cells. BMMNCs have demonstrated neurogenic potential and exhibit various paracrine effects like angiogenesis, upregulation of anti-inflammatory cytokines, secreting neurotrophic factors and growth factors, bring about immune modulation and stimulate resident stem cells. While the less invasive systemic routes, lead to dilution of the cells reaching the target organ, due to filtration of cells in various organs like liver, spleen, kidneys and lungs; more invasive routes like intra-spinal routes pose risk of procedure related adverse effect. Intra-thecal delivery therefore ensures delivery of maximum cells at the site of the injury with relatively reduced risk of procedure related adverse effects.

6.1.4.1 Role of rehabilitation

It is important that regenerative therapies are complimented with rehabilitative therapies like physiotherapy, occupational therapy, aquatic therapy, speech therapy, psychological intervention and nutritional advice. Regular goal-oriented rehabilitation provides neuroprotective, my protective, anti-inflammatory, antioxidant and neoangiogenic effects on a systemic level which resonate with the paracrine effects of cell therapy and compliment the effect of cell therapy. It is also believed that exercise can contribute to sub-granular and sub-ventricular neurogenesis. Neurogenesis consists of various processes. While differentiation, migration and axonal guidance are independent of physical activity synaptic pruning and plasticity is dependent of physical activity and therefore rehabilitation plays a pivotal role in enhancing this. Therefore, we prescribe a regime of multidisciplinary rehabilitation to be followed at home after the cell transplantation (**Figure 2**).

6.1.5 Adverse effects

This protocol is safe without any major adverse effects. We have so far treated more than 800 patients with spinal cord injury and none of the patients have exhibited any major irreversible adverse effects. A small percentage of patients have shown some minor procedure related adverse effects in SCI which are headache, pain at the site of injection, nausea and vomiting. These are usually self-limiting or can be completely relieved with minor medical intervention.

6.2 Published results

6.2.1 Thoracolumbar spinal cord injury

A detailed analysis of chronic thoracolumbar SCI patients who underwent intrathecal administration of autologous bone marrow mononuclear cells followed by neurorehabilitation was conducted [84]. The study sample included 110 thoracolumbar SCI patients. The outcome was recorded at a mean follow up of

2 years ± 1 month. The outcome measures were functional independence measure (FIM) score, American Spinal Injury Association scale (ASIA) and detailed neurological assessment. Data were statistically analyzed using McNemar's Test to establish significance between the change in symptoms and the intervention.

A total of 100 out of 110 (91%) patients showed improvements. Improvement in trunk control was observed in 95.6% cases, bladder management in 33% with respect to shift from indwelling and condom catheter to self-intermittent catheterization, partial sensory recovery in 27% and reduction of spasticity in 26%. All the patients showed improvement in postural hypotension. 38% wheelchair bound patients started walking with assistance. Functionally, 27% showed improved activities of daily living (ADLs) and 53.6% showed a positive change in FIM score. About 10% cases showed a shift in ASIA scale. A statistically significant association of these symptomatic improvements with the cell therapy intervention was established using McNemar's Test. On electrophysiological studies, 2 showed improvement and 1 showed change in functional MRI [79] (**Figure 6**, **Tables 1** and **2**).

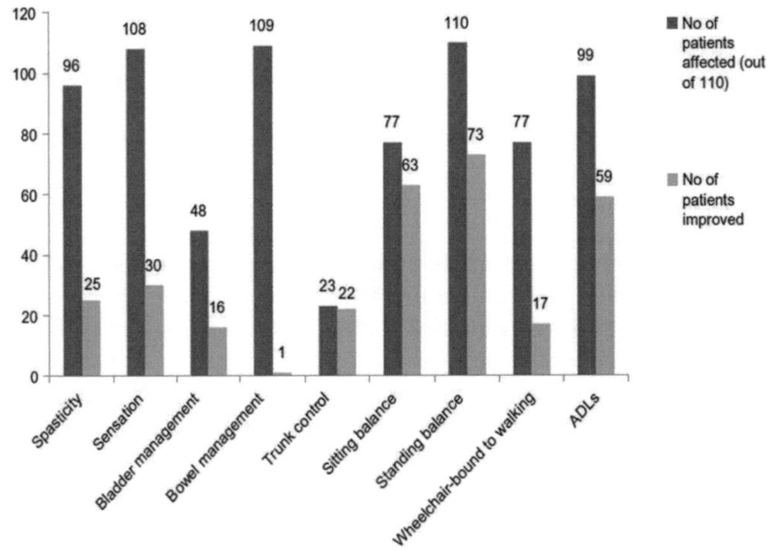

Figure 6.
*Symptomatic improvements in patients with spinal cord injury after stem cell therapy. The X-axis denotes symptoms presented in the patient population and the Y-axis denotes the number of patients. (ADLs—activities of daily living) (**Tables 1** and **2**).*

Symptom/function	Affected patients (n of 110)	Patients improved (n)	Chi-square value†	P value#
Spasticity	96	25	23.04	<0.0001
Sensation	108	30	28.033	<0.0001
Bladder management	48	16	14.06	0.0002
Bowel management	109	1	0	1.000*
Trunk control	23	22	20.045	<0.0001
Sitting balance	77	63	61.016	<0.0001
Standing balance	110	73	70.014	<0.0001
Wheelchair-bound to walking	77	17	15.059	0.0001
ADLs	99	59	57.017	<0.0001

Notes: #Significant at $P \leq 0.05$; †Chi-square value at one degree of freedom; *P value insignificant for improvement in bowel management.
Abbreviation: ADLs, activities of daily living.

Table 1.
Statistical significance for each symptomatic/functional change using McNemar's test.

(A)	Nerve/sites	Amplitude 2–4 mV (before)	Amplitude 2–4 mV (after)
Patient 1	R tibial (knee)-AH ankle	3.5	5.4
	R tibial (knee)-AH knee	2.7	5.1
	L tibial (knee)-AH ankle	4.1	5.7
	R tibial (knee)-gastrocnemius knee	7.2	14.8
	L tibial (knee)-gastrocnemius knee	10.2	11.7
Patient 2	L common peroneal-EDB ankle	0.8	3.0
	R common peroneal – tibialis anterior, fibular head	1.6	3.4
	L common peroneal – tibialis anterior, fibular head	1.8	4.3
	R tibial (knee)-AH ankle	7.0	8.0
	L tibial (knee)-AH ankle	7.9	8.3
	R tibial (knee)-gastrocnemius knee	6.2	18.7
	L tibial (knee)-gastrocnemius knee	2.5	17.2
(B)	**Functional MRI (before)**	**Functional MRI (after)**	
Patient 1	No activity in the pre and post central gyri	Activation in the right precentral gyrus	

Abbreviations: AH, abductor hallucis; EDB, extensor digitorum brevis; MRI, magnetic resonance imaging; R, right; L, left.

Table 2.
Objective improvements evident on electromyography (A) and functional magnetic resonance imaging (B) after stem cell therapy in selected patients.

6.2.2 Cervical SCI

A detailed analysis of chronic cervical SCI patients who underwent intrathecal administration of autologous bone marrow mononuclear cells followed by neurorehabilitation was conducted [85]. This study includes 50 patients of chronic cervical SCI. The outcome was recorded at a mean follow up of 2 years ± 1 month. The outcome measures were functional independence measure (FIM) score, American Spinal Injury Association scale (ASIA) and detailed neurological assessment. Data were statistically analyzed using McNemar's Test to establish significance between the change in symptoms and the intervention. 37 out of 50 (74%) showed improvements. Sensation recovery was observed in 26% cases, improved trunk control in 22.4%, spasticity reduction in 20% and bladder sensation recovery in 14.2%. All the 50 cases had improvement in postural hypotension. 12.24% wheelchair bound patients started walking with assistance. Functionally, 20.4% patients showed improved ADLs and 48% showed a positive change in FIM score. 6% cases showed a shift in ASIA scale. A statistical analysis using McNemar's test established a significant association of these symptoms with the intervention [89]. No major side effects were noted in the duration of 2 years in both the studies. A better outcome was observed in thoracolumbar injury as compared to the cervical injury suggesting that the level of SCI greatly influences the recovery of the patient (**Tables 3–5**). Both studies demonstrated statistically significant clinical and functional outcome (**Figure 7**).

Symptom	No. of patients affected	No. of patients improved	McNemars test value	P value
Spasticity	49	9	7.11111	*0.00766
Sensation	51	11	9.09091	*0.00257
Bladder Sensation	34	7	5.14286	*0.02334
Upper Limb Strength	50	26	24.03846	*<0.000001
Sitting Balance	32	28	26.03571	*<0.000001
Standing Balance	56	27	25.03704	*<0.000001
Walking Balance	56	8	6.125	*0.01333
Trunk Stability	13	12	10.08333	*0.0015
Trunk muscle strength	9	7	5.14286	*0.02334
Postural Hypotension	11	11	9.09091	*0.00257

*significant at p value ≤ 0.05

Table 3.
McNemar's test: table demonstrating the statistical analysis for each symptomatic improvement in cervical SCI using McNemar's test.

Factors		Percentage improvements
Age	<18 yrs	100%
	18-35 yrs	41%
	>35 yrs	42%
Cause of Trauma	RTA	37.20%
	Non-RTA	30%
Chronicity	1-3 yrs	47.82%
	3-5 yrs	33.33%
	>5 yrs	44.44%
Rehabilitation	Done	36.84%
	Not Done	55.55%

Table 4.
Percentage analysis of improvements: table demonstrating a detailed analysis of various factors and the improvements.

Symptoms improved	Cervical SCI	Thoracolumbar SCI
Spasticity	18.37%	26%
Sensation	21.57%	28%
Bladder Sensation	20.59%	33%
Bowel Sensation	5.66%	0.9%
Sitting Balance	87.50%	81.81%
Standing Balance	48.21%	66.36
Trunk Stability	92.31%	95.65%
Postural Hypotension	100.00%	100%

Table 5.
Comparison between cervical SCI and thoracolumbar SCI: table comparing the outcome of cell transplantation in cervical SCI and thoracolumbar SCI.

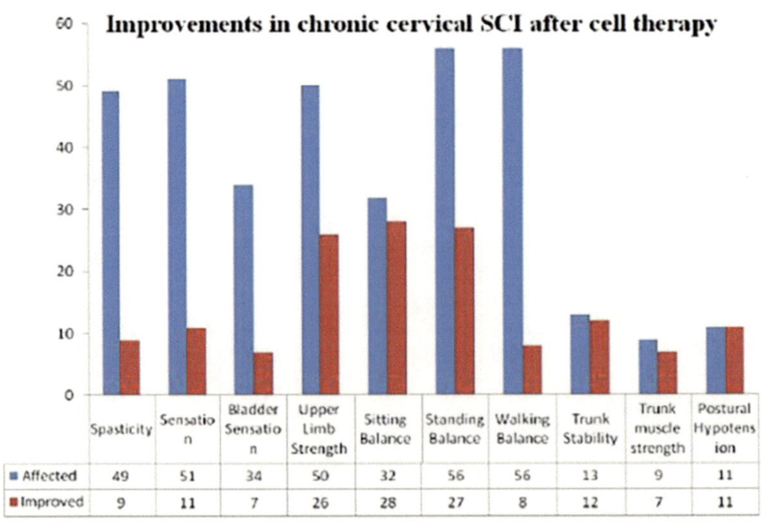

Figure 7.
Graph demonstrating symptomatic improvements in chronic cervical SCI patients after cell therapy.

6.2.3 Objective assessment using neuroimaging

A case study of a 32-year-old man with chronic thoracic complete spinal cord injury treated with intrathecal administration of autologous bone marrow mononuclear cells with standard rigorous neurorehabilitation showed improved clinical outcome without any adverse effect [93]. Follow up assessment conducted at 3- and 7-months post treatment showed improvements in motor activities, ambulation, bed mobilities, transfers and bladder management. Spinal cord independence measure (SCIM) improved from 27 to 64/100 and functional improvement measure (FIM) improved from 64 to 83 suggesting significant functional gain.

Brain functional magnetic resonance imaging (fMRI) shows patterns of cortical activation in response to attempted motor task. In chronic spinal cord injury corticospinal tract neurons undergo retrograde degeneration. Therefore, the activation of the cortical areas is reduced in response to injury. Brain fMRI can thus be used to assess the outcome of the therapy. Post treatment fMRI in these patients showed activation of multiple regions in the sensory and associated areas, which was absent pre-treatment providing evidence for improved neural activation (**Figure 8**).

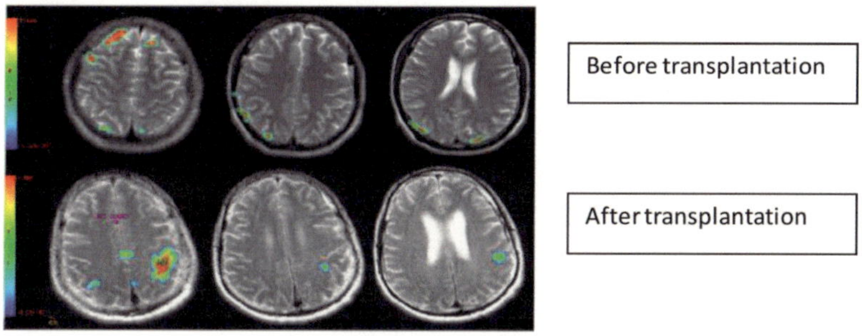

Figure 8.
fMRI images showing improved activation of sensorimotor and associated areas post transplantation.

6.3 Unpublished data

We analyzed 300 patients with chronic thoracic and cervical spinal cord injury and noted that 96.2% of the patients showed clinical improvements. The improvements were classified as mild, moderate or significant based on how many

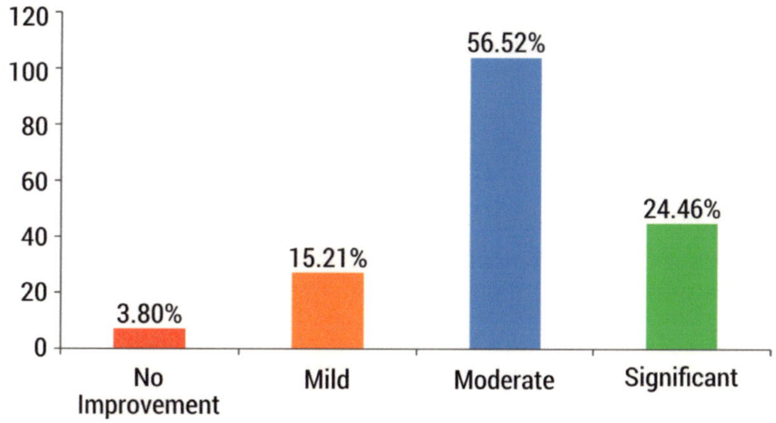

Figure 9.
Clinical outcome in patients with SCI post cell treatment.

symptoms showed improvements (3 symptoms—mild improvement, 4–6 symptoms—moderate improvement and more than 6 symptoms—significant improvement) majority of the patients showed moderate improvements (**Figure 9**).

Symptomatic analysis of these patients showed reduction in spasticity, sensory motor recovery, recovery of bladder sensation, increased functional independence while performing ADLS, improved balance and ambulation (**Figure 10**).

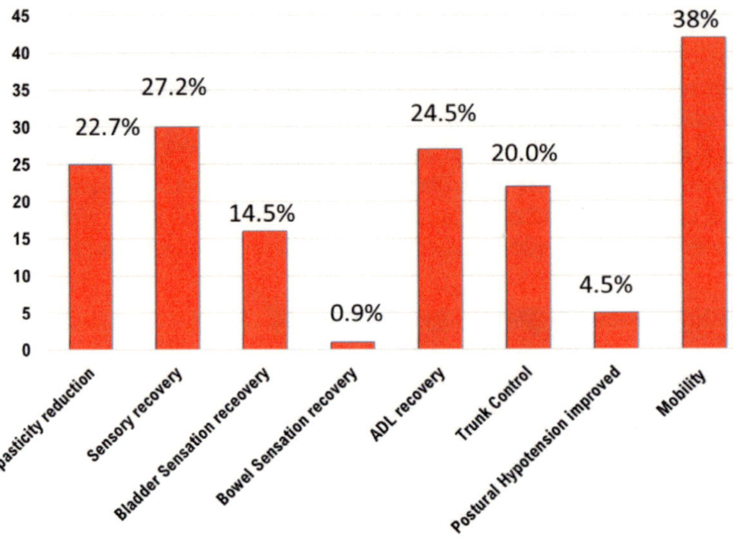

Figure 10.
Symptomatic improvements in patients with SCI post cell therapy.

7. Limitations and future directions

Currently little objective evidence is available to show the regeneration of spinal cord and increased connectivity of spinal tracts. Enhanced radio imaging tools are required for better visualization of the outcome.

Although various cells and routes of administration have been explored an optimum cell type and route of administration remain elusive due to heterogeneity of research protocols, sample size, treatment regimen and lack of multi-centric high-quality studies. Comparison between different protocols is required to be carried out using rigorous methodology to identify an optimum clinical protocol that yields maximum recovery.

It takes about 6 months to generate iPSCs from autologous somatic cells and almost a year to test the safety of cells for transplantation, this combines with risks associated with iPSCs including genetic and epigenetic abnormalities, tumorigenicity and immunogenicity related to cell trans-plantation has prevented their clinical translation so far [94–96]. Advent in iPSC technology and its clinical translation is the future direction for medical sciences.

8. Conclusion

Spinal cord injury is a devastating and disabling neurological disorder with no definite cure. Several treatment strategies are being explored for improved clinical outcome especially for chronic injuries. Stem cell therapy is a promising treatment modality. Use of stem cells for the treatment of spinal cord injury is safe and improves neurological as well as functional outcome. With the available evidence autologous multipotent stem cells like bone marrow derived mononuclear cells show positive clinical outcomes with no adverse effects. Factors like level of injury, time since injury, concomitant disorders and rigor of neurorehabilitation can influence the outcome of the cell treatment.

Lot of evidence has been generated over the last decade demonstrating the benefits of using stem cells to improve sensory-motor function, functional independence of the patients and quality of life. Stem cell therapy helps to reduce the complications post spinal cord injury due to their positive effect. Although it does not provide a complete cure at the moment, it certainly holds the potential to improve functional independence and quality of life. It is important to supplement stem cell therapy with current treatments and rehabilitation for optimum clinical improvement.

Author details

Alok Sharma, Hemangi Sane, Nandini Gokulchandran, Prerna Badhe, Amruta Paranjape*, Pooja Kulkarni and Vivek Nair
NeuroGen Brain and Spine Institute, Navi Mumbai, India

*Address all correspondence to: amrutap.neurogen@gmail.com

References

[1] Silva NA, Sousa N, Reis RL. From basics to clinical: A comprehensive review on spinal cord injury. Progress in Neurobiology. 2014;**114**:25-57

[2] Wyndaele M, Wyndaele JJ. Incidence, prevalence and epidemiology of spinal cord injury: What learns a worldwide literature survey? Spinal Cord. 2006;**44**(9):523

[3] Lee BB, Cripps RA, Fitzharris M, et al. The global map for traumatic spinal cord injury epidemiology: Update, global incidence rate. Spinal Cord. 2011;**52**(2):110-116

[4] Zhao H, Sun QL, Duan LJ, Yang YD, Gao YS, Zhao DY, et al. Is cell transplantation a reliable therapeutic strategy for spinal cord injury in clinical practice? A systematic review and meta-analysis from 22 clinical controlled trials. European Spine Journal. 2019;**21**:1092-1112

[5] Hurlbert RJ, Hadley MN, Walters BC, et al. Pharmacological therapy for acute spinal cord injury. Neurosurgery. 2015;**76**:S71-S83

[6] Miller SM. Methylprednisolone in acute spinal cord injury: A tarnished standard. Journal of Neurosurgical Anesthesiology. 2008;**20**(2):140-142

[7] Yue JK, Chan AK, Winkler EA, Upadhyayula PS, Readdy WJ, Dhall SS. A review and update on the guidelines for the acute management of cervical spinal cord injury—Part II. Journal of Neurosurgical Sciences. 2016;**60**(3):367-384

[8] Ditunno JF, Cardenas DD, Formal C, Dalal K. Advances in the rehabilitation management of acute spinal cord injury. Handbook of Clinical Neurology. 2012;**109**:181-195

[9] Marino G, Rosso F, Ferdinando P, et al. Growth and endothelial differentiation of adipose stem cells on polycaprolactone. Journal of Biomedical Materials Research. Part A. 2012;**100**(3):543-548

[10] Barbarisi M, Marino G, Armenia E. mUse of polycaprolactone (PCL) as scaffolds for the regeneration of nerve tissue. Journal of Biomedical Materials Research. Part A. 2015;**103**(5):1755-1760

[11] Sahni V, Kessler JA. Stem cell therapies for spinal cord injury. Nature Reviews. Neurology. 2010;**6**(7):363-372

[12] Ruff CA, Wilcox JT, Fehlings MG. Cell-based transplantation strategies to promote plasticity following spinal cord injury. Experimental Neurology. 2012;**235**(1):78-90

[13] Frantz S. Embryonic stem cell pioneer Geron exits field, cuts losses. Nature Biotechnology. 2012;**30**:12-13

[14] Geffner LF, Santacruz P, Izurieta M, Flor L, Maldonado B, Auad AH, et al. Administration of autologous bone marrow stem cells into spinal cord injury patients via multiple routes is safe and improves their quality of life: Comprehensive case studies. Cell Transplantation. 2008;**17**(12):1277-1293

[15] El-Kheir WA, Gabr H, Awad MR, Ghannam O, Barakat Y, Farghali HA, et al. Autologous bone marrow-derived cell therapy combined with physical therapy induces functional improvement in chronic spinal cord injury patients. Cell Transplantation. 2014;**23**(6):729-745

[16] Zhou Q, Zhang SZ, Xu RX, Xu K. Neural stem cell transplantation and postoperative management: Report of 70 cases. Di Yi Jun Yi Da Xue Xue Bao. 2004;**24**(10):1207-1209

[17] Moviglia GA, Fernandez Viña R, Brizuela JA, et al. Combined protocol of cell therapy for chronic spinal cord injury. Report on the electrical and functional recovery of two patients. Cytotherapy. 2006;**8**(3):202-209

[18] Knoller N, Auerbach G, Fulga V, et al. Clinical experience using incubated autologous macrophages as a treatment for complete spinal cord injury: Phase I study results. Journal of Neurosurgery. Spine. 2005;**3**(3):173-181

[19] Cristante F, Barros-Filho TEP, Barros-Filho TEP. Stem cells in the treatment of chronic spinal cord injury: Evaluation of somatosensitive evoked potentials in 39 patients. Spinal Cord. 2009;**47**(10):733-738

[20] Ichim TE, Solano F, Lara F, et al. Feasibility of combination allogeneic stem cell therapy for spinal cord injury: A case report. International Archives of Medicine. 2010;**3**:30

[21] Lima P, Escada J, Pratas-Vital J, et al. Olfactory mucosal autografts and rehabilitation for chronic traumatic spinal cord injury. Neurorehabilitation and Neural Repair. 2010;**24**(1):10-22

[22] Ra JC, Shin IS, Kim SH, Kang SK, Kang BC, Lee HY, et al. Safety of intravenous infusion of human adipose tissue-derived mesenchymal stem cells in animals and humans. Stem Cells and Development. 2011;**20**(8):1297-1308

[23] Raisman G. Repair of spinal cord injury by transplantation of olfactory ensheathing cells. Comptes Rendus Biologies. 2007;**330**(6-7):557-560

[24] Huang H, Xi H, Chen L, Zhang F, Liu Y. Long-term outcome of olfactory ensheathing cell therapy for patients with complete chronic spinal cord injury. Cell Transplantation. 2012;**21**(Suppl 1):S23-S31

[25] Saberi H, Firouzi M, Habibi Z, Moshayedi P, Aghayan HR, Arjmand B, et al. Safety of intramedullary Schwann cell transplantation for post rehabilitation spinal cord injuries: 2-year follow-up of 33 cases. Journal of Neurosurgery. Spine. 2011;**15**(5):515-525

[26] Yazdani SO, Hafizi M, Zali AR, Atashi A, Ashrafi F, Seddighi AS, et al. Safety and possible outcome assessment of autologous Schwann cell and bone marrow mesenchymal stromal cell co-transplantation for treatment of patients with chronic spinal cord injury. Cytotherapy. 2013;**15**(7):782-791

[27] Sun T, Ye C, Zhang Z, Wu J, Huang H. Co transplantation of olfactory ensheathing cells and Schwann cells combined with treadmill training promotes functional recovery in rats with contused spinal cords. Cell Transplantation. 2013;**22**(Suppl 1):S27-S38

[28] Chen L, Huang H, Xi H, Zhang F, Liu Y, Chen D, et al. A prospective randomized double-blind clinical trial using a combination of olfactory ensheathing cells and Schwann cells for the treatment of chronic complete spinal cord injuries. Cell Transplantation. 2014;**23**(Suppl 1):S35-S44

[29] Al-Zoubi A, Jafar E, Jamous M, Al-Twal F, Al-Bakheet S, Zalloum M, et al. Transplantation of purified autologous leukapheresis-derived CD34+ and CD133+ stem cells for patients with chronic spinal cord injuries: Long-term evaluation of safety and efficacy. Cell Transplantation. 2014;**23**(Suppl 1):S25-S34

[30] Cheng H, Liu X, Hua R, Dai G, Wang X, Gao J, et al. Clinical observation of umbilical cord mesenchymal stem cell transplantation in treatment for sequelae of thoracolumbar spinal cord injury. Journal of Translational Medicine. 2014;**12**:253

[31] Syková E, Jendelová P, Urdzíková L, Lesný P, Hejcl A. Bone marrow stem cells and polymer hydrogels-two strategies for spinal cord injury repair. Cellular and Molecular Neurobiology. 2006;**26**(7-8):1113-1129

[32] Syková E, Homola A, Mazanec R, et al. Autologous bone marrow transplantation in patients with subacute and chronic spinal cord injury. Cell Transplantation. 2006;**15**:1-100

[33] Chernykh R, Stupak VV, Muradov GM, et al. Application of autologous bone marrow stem cells in the therapy of spinal cord injury patients. Bulletin of Experimental Biology and Medicine. 2007;**143**(4):543-547

[34] Frasch M. Dedifferentiation, redifferentiation, and trans differentiation of striated muscles during regeneration and development. Current Topics in Developmental Biology. 2016;**116**:331-355

[35] Jopling C, Boue S, Belmonte JC. Dedifferentiation, trans-differentiation and reprogramming: Three routes to regeneration. Nature Reviews. Molecular Cell Biology. 2011;**12**(2):79

[36] Baker CL, Pera MF. Capturing totipotent stem cells. Cell Stem Cell. 2018;**22**(1):25-34

[37] Singh VK, Saini A, Kalsan M, Kumar N, Chandra R. Describing the stem cell potency: The various methods of functional assessment and in silico diagnostics. Frontiers in Cell and Development Biology. 2016;**4**:134

[38] Alizadeh A, Dyck SM, Karimi-Abdolrezaee S. Traumatic spinal cord injury: An overview of pathophysiology, models and acute injury mechanisms. Frontiers in Neurology. 2019;**10**:282

[39] Keirstead HS, Nistor G, Bernal G, Totoiu M, Cloutier F, Sharp K, et al. Human embryonic stem cell-derived oligodendrocyte progenitor cell transplants remyelinate and restore locomotion after spinal cord injury. The Journal of Neuroscience. 2005;**25**(19):4694-4705

[40] Karimi-Abdolrezaee S, Eftekharpour E, Wang J, Morshead CM, Fehlings MG. Delayed transplantation of adult neural precursor cells promotes remyelination and functional neurological recovery after spinal cord injury. The Journal of Neuroscience. 2006;**26**(13):3377-3389

[41] Dasari VR, Spomar DG, Gondi CS, Sloffer CA, Saving KL, Gujrati M, et al. Axonal remyelination by cord blood stem cells after spinal cord injury. Journal of Neurotrauma. 2007;**24**(2):391-410

[42] Akiyama Y, Radtke C, Kocsis JD. Remyelination of the rat spinal cord by transplantation of identified bone marrow stromal cells. The Journal of Neuroscience. 2002;**22**(15):6623-6630

[43] Pineau I, Lacroix S. Proinflammatory cytokine synthesis in the injured mouse spinal cord: Multiphasic expression pattern and identification of the cell types involved. The Journal of Comparative Neurology. 2007;**500**:267-285

[44] Kettenmann H, Hanisch UK, Noda M, Verkhratsky A. Physiology of microglia. Physiological Reviews. 2001;**91**:461-553

[45] Oyinbo CA. Secondary injury mechanisms in traumatic spinal cord injury: A nugget of this multiply cascade. Acta Neurobiologiae Experimentalis (Wars). 2011;**71**:281-299

[46] Kong X, Gao J. Macrophage polarization: A key event in the secondary phase of acute spinal cord injury. Journal of Cellular and Molecular Medicine. 2017;**21**:941-954. DOI: 10.1111/jcmm.13034

[47] Saporta S, Kim JJ, Willing AE, Fu ES, Davis CD, Sanberg PR. Human umbilical cord blood stem cells infusion in spinal cord injury: Engraftment and beneficial influence on behavior. Journal of Hematotherapy & Stem Cell Research. 2003;**12**(3):271-278

[48] Urdzíková L, Růžička J, LaBagnara M, Kárová K, Kubinová Š, Jiráková K, et al. Human mesenchymal stem cells modulate inflammatory cytokines after spinal cord injury in rat. International Journal of Molecular Sciences. 2014;**15**(7):11275-11293

[49] Kim Y, Jo SH, Kim WH, Kweon OK. Antioxidant and anti-inflammatory effects of intravenously injected adipose derived mesenchymal stem cells in dogs with acute spinal cord injury. Stem Cell Research & Therapy. 2015;**6**(1):229

[50] Cheng Z, Zhu W, Cao K, Wu F, Li J, Wang G, et al. Anti-inflammatory mechanism of neural stem cell transplantation in spinal cord injury. International Journal of Molecular Sciences. 2016;**17**(9):1380

[51] Urdzíková L, Jendelová P, Glogarová K, Burian M, Hájek M, Syková E. Transplantation of bone marrow stem cells as well as mobilization by granulocyte-colony stimulating factor promotes recovery after spinal cord injury in rats. Journal of Neurotrauma. 2006;**23**(9):1379-1391

[52] Kumagai G, Okada Y, Yamane J, Nagoshi N, Kitamura K, Mukaino M, et al. Roles of ES cell-derived gliogenic neural stem/progenitor cells in functional recovery after spinal cord injury. PLoS ONE. 2009;**4**(11):e7706

[53] Kim HM, Hwang DH, Lee JE, Kim SU, Kim BG. Ex vivo VEGF delivery by neural stem cells enhances proliferation of glial progenitors, angiogenesis, and tissue sparing after spinal cord injury. PLoS ONE. 2009;**4**(3):e4987

[54] Quertainmont R, Cantinieaux D, Botman O, Sid S, Schoenen J, Franzen R. Mesenchymal stem cell graft improves recovery after spinal cord injury in adult rats through neurotrophic and pro-angiogenic actions. PLoS ONE. 2012;**7**(6):e39500

[55] Ogawa Y, Sawamoto K, Miyata T, Miyao S, Watanabe M, Nakamura M, et al. Transplantation of in vitro-expanded fetal neural progenitor cells results in neurogenesis and functional recovery after spinal cord contusion injury in adult rats. Journal of Neuroscience Research. 2002;**69**(6):925-933

[56] Deng YB, Liu XG, Liu ZG, Liu XL, Liu Y, Zhou GQ. Implantation of BM mesenchymal stem cells into injured spinal cord elicits de novo neurogenesis and functional recovery: Evidence from a study in rhesus monkeys. Cytotherapy. 2006;**8**(3):210-214

[57] Lu P, Jones LL, Snyder EY, Tuszynski MH. Neural stem cells constitutively secrete neurotrophic factors and promote extensive host axonal growth after spinal cord injury. Experimental Neurology. 2003;**181**(2):115-129

[58] Smith AG. Embryo-derived stem cells: Of mice and men. Annual Review of Cell and Developmental Biology. 2001;**17**:435-462. DOI: 10.1146/annurev.cellbio.17.1.435

[59] Nistor GI, Totoiu MO, Haque N, Carpenter MK, Keirstead HS. Human embryonic stem cells differentiate into oligodendrocytes in high purity and myelinate after spinal cord transplantation. Glia. 2005;**49**:385-396

[60] Cloutier F, Siegenthaler MM, Nistor G, Keirstead HS. Transplantation of human embryonic stem cell-derived oligodendrocyte progenitors into rat t spinal cord injuries does not cause harm. Regenerative Medicine. 2006;**1**:469-479

[61] Salewski RP, Mitchell RA, Shen C, Fehlings MG. Transplantation of neural stem cells clonally derived from embryonic stem cells promotes recovery after murine spinal cord injury. Stem Cells and Development. 2015;**24**:36-50

[62] Faulkner J, Keirstead HS. Human embryonic stem cell-derived oligodendrocyte progenitors for the treatment of spinal cord injury. Transplant Immunology. 2005;**15**:131-142

[63] Zhang YW, Denham J, Thies RS. Oligodendrocyte progenitor cells derived from human embryonic stem cells express neurotrophic factors. Stem Cells. 2006;**15**:943-952

[64] Tetzlaff W, Okon EB, Karimi-Abdolrezaee S, Hill CE, Sparling JS, Plemel JR, et al. A systematic review of cellular transplantation therapies for spinal cord injury. Journal of Neurotrauma. 2011;**28**:1611-1682

[65] Salewski RP, Mitchell RA, Li L, Shen C, Milekovskaia M, Nagy A, et al. Transplantation of induced pluripotent stem cell-derived neural stem cells mediate functional recovery following thoracic spinal cord injury through remyelination of axons. Stem Cells Translational Medicine. 2015;**4**:743-754

[66] Shende P, Subedi M. Pathophysiology, mechanisms and applications of mesenchymal stem cells for the treatment of spinal cord injury. Biomedicine & Pharmacotherapy. 2017;**91**:693-706

[67] Nagoshi N, Okano H. Applications of induced pluripotent stem cell technologies in spinal cord injury. Journal of Neurochemistry. 2017;**141**:848-860

[68] Fujimoto Y, Abematsu M, Falk A, Tsujimura K, Sanosaka T, Juliandi B, et al. Treatment of a mouse model of spinal cord injury by transplantation of human induced pluripotent stem cell-derived long-term self-renewing neuroepithelial-like stem cells. Stem Cells. 2012;**30**:1163-1173

[69] Kobayashi Y, Okada Y, Itakura G, Iwai H, Nishimura S, Yasuda A, et al. Pre-evaluated safe human iPSC-derived neural stem cells promote functional recovery after spinal cord injury in common marmoset without tumorigenicity. PLoS ONE. 2012;**7**:e52787

[70] Nutt SE, Chang EA, Suhr ST, Schlosser LO, Mondello SE, Moritz CT, et al. Caudalized human iPSC-derived neural progenitor cells produce neurons and glia but fail to restore function in an early chronic spinal cord injury model. Experimental Neurology. 2013;**248**:491-503

[71] Amemori T, Ruzicka J, RomanyukN,Jhanwar-UniyalM,SykovaE, Jendelova P. Comparison of intraspinal and intrathecal implantation of induced pluripotent stem cell-derived neural precursors for the treatment of spinal cord injury in rats. Stem Cell Research & Therapy. 2015;**6**:257

[72] Hayashi K, Hashimoto M, Koda M, Naito AT, Murata A, Okawa A et al. Increase of sensitivity to mechanical stimulus after transplantation of murine induced pluripotent stem cell-derived astro astrocytes in a rat spinal cord injury model. Journal of Neurosurgery Spine. Dec 2011;**15**(6):582-593

[73] Rabinovich SS, Seledtsov VI, Poveschenko OV. Transplantation treatment of spinal cord injury patients. Biomedicine & Pharmacotherapy. 2003;**57**(9):428-433

[74] Feron F, Perry C, Cochrane J, Licina P, Nowitzke A, Urquhart S, et al. Autologous olfactory ensheathing cell transplantation in human spinal cord injury. Brain. 2005;**128**(12):2951-2960

[75] Mackay-Sim F, Féron J, Cochrane J, et al. Autologous olfactory ensheathing cell transplantation in human paraplegia: A 3-year clinical trial. Brain. 2008;**131**(9):2376-2386

[76] Subbaiah GPV, Adavi V, Chelluri LK, Laxman S, Ratnakar KS, Gopal PBN, et al. Preliminary report on the safety, efficacy and functional recovery of spinal cord injury with autologous bone marrow derived mesenchymal stem cells—A clinical trial. The Internet Journal of Spine Surgery. 2009;**5**(1)

[77] Jarocha D, Milczarek O, Kawecki Z, Wendrychowicz A, Kwiatkowski S, Majka M. Preliminary study of autologous bone marrow nucleated cells transplantation in children with spinal cord injury. Stem Cells Translational Medicine. Mar 2014;**3**(3):395-404

[78] Ha Y, Yoon SH, Park SR. Treatment of complete spinal cord injury patients receiving autologous bone marrow cell transplantation and bone marrow stimulation with granulocyte macrophage-colony stimulating factor—Report of three cases. Journal of Korean Neurosurgical Association. 2004;**35**:459-464

[79] Park HC, Shim YS, Ha Y, et al. Treatment of complete spinal cord injury patients by autologous bone marrow cell transplantation and Administration of granulocyte-macrophage colony stimulating factor. Tissue Engineering. 2005;**11**(5-6):913-922

[80] Deda H, Inci MC, Kürekçi AE, Kayihan K, Ozgün E, Ustünsoy GE, et al. Treatment of chronic spinal cord injured patients with autologous bone marrow-derived hematopoietic stem cell transplantation: 1-year follow-up. Cytotherapy. 2008;**10**(6):565-574

[81] Frolov AA, Bryukhovetskiy AS Effects of hematopoietic autologous stem cell transplantation to the chronically injured human spinal cord evaluated by motor and somatosensory evoked potentials methods. Cell Transplantation. 2012;**21**(Suppl 1): S49-S55

[82] Dai G, Liu X, Zhang Z, Yang Z, Dai Y, Xu R. Transplantation of autologous bone marrow mesenchymal stem cells in the treatment of complete and chronic cervical spinal cord injury. Brain Research. 2013;**1533**:73-79

[83] Jiang PC, Xiong WP, Wang G, Ma C, Yao WQ, Kendell SF, et al. A clinical trial report of autologous bone marrow-derived mesenchymal stem cell transplantation in patients with spinal cord injury. Experimental and Therapeutic Medicine. 2013;**6**(1):140-146

[84] Sharma A, Gokulchandran N, Sane H, Badhe P, Kulkarni P, Lohia M, et al. Detailed analysis of the clinical effects of cell therapy for thoracolumbar spinal cord injury: An original study. Journal of Neurorestoratology. 2013;**1**:13-22

[85] Sharma A, Sane H, Gokulchandran N, Kulkarni P, Thomas N, et al. Role of autologous bone marrow mononuclear cells in chronic cervical spinal cord injury—A Long-term follow up study. Journal of Neurological Disorders. 2013;**1**:138

[86] Abdelaziz OS. Feasibility, safety, and efficacy of directly transplanting autologous adult bone marrow stem cells in patients with chronic traumatic dorsal cord injury: A pilot clinical study. Neurosurgery Quarterly. 2010;**20**(3):216-226

[87] Saberi H, Moshayedi P, Aghayan H-R, et al. Treatment of chronic thoracic spinal cord injury patients with autologous Schwann cell transplantation: An interim report on safety considerations and possible

outcomes. Neuroscience Letters. 2008;**443**(1):46-50

[88] Park JH, Kim DY, Sung IY, et al. Long-term results of spinal cord injury therapy using mesenchymal stem cells derived from bone marrow in humans. Neurosurgery. 2012;**70**(5):1238-1247

[89] Saito F, Nakatani T, Iwase M, et al. Spinal cord injury treatment with intrathecal autologous bone marrow stromal cell transplantation: The first clinical trial case report. The Journal of Trauma. 2008;**64**(1):53-59

[90] Pal R, Venkataramana NK, Bansal A, et al. Ex vivo expanded autologous bone marrow-derived mesenchymal stromal cells in human spinal cord injury/ paraplegia: A pilot clinical study. Cytotherapy. 2009;**11**(7):897-911

[91] Kumar A, Kumar SR, Narayanan R, Arul K, Baskaran M. Autologous bone marrow derived mononuclear cell therapy for spinal cord injury: A phase I/ II clinical safety and primary efficacy data. Experimental and Clinical Transplantation. 2009;**7**(4):241-248

[92] Callera F, do Nascimento RX. Delivery of autologous bone marrow precursor cells into the spinal cord via lumbar puncture technique in patients with spinal cord injury: A preliminary safety study. Experimental Hematology. 2006;**34**(2):130-131

[93] Alok S, Prerna B, Suhasini P, Hemangi S, Samson N, Pooja K, et al. Functional recovery and functional magnetic resonance imaging changes following cellular therapy in a case of chronic complete spinal cord injury. Current Trends in Clinical & Medical Imaging. 2017;**1**(4):555566

[94] Okano H, Nakamura M, Yoshida K, Okada Y, Tsuji O, Nori S, et al. Steps toward safe cell therapy using induced pluripotent stem cells. Circulation Research. 2013;**112**:523-533

[95] Nishimura S, Yasuda A, Iwai H, et al. Time-dependent changes in the microenvironment of injured spinal cord affects the therapeutic potential of neural stem cell transplantation for spinal cord injury. Molecular Brain. 2013;**6**:3

[96] Iwai H, Shimada H, Nishimura S, et al. Allogeneic neural stem/progenitor cells derived from embryonic stem cells promote functional recovery after transplantation into injured spinal cord of nonhuman primates. Stem Cells Translational Medicine. 2015;**4**:708-719